INDEX OF DIFFERENTIATIONS FOR COMMONLY USED HERB FORMULATIONS

ISBN: 0-941942-15-5

Printed in Taiwan, R.O.C.

CONTENTS

Notice

The following is a summary description of some of the natural herbal formulas widely used throughout Asia. The information compiled from traditional medical texts and from the observations of modern authorities on Chinese medicine is presented here for its educational value and should not be used for diagnosis, treatment, or prevention of disease without the advice of a Chinese physician or other medical authority.

Preface

Although Chinese medicine has existed for 5,000 years and been used by more than one billion people in Asia (including Korea, Japan, Taiwan, and Hong Kong), it remained unknown to the Western world for many centuries because of its different theory and practice. Since former President Richard Nixon visited China in 1972, acupuncture has become the best known facet of Chinese medicine. Indeed acupuncture itself has gained acceptance, but the Western medical and scientific community has never considered seriously the medical tradition and culture from which this technique sprang. To introduce more traditional Chinese medicine to the Western world, I founded the Oriental Healing Arts Institute (OHAI) in 1976, with a view to translating traditional Chinese medical texts into English and other languages and presenting the Chinese cultural medical tradition. So far we have succeeded in publishing fifteen books and fifty issues of the Bulletin, attracting public attention to the art of medicine from a different viewpoint.

The basis of the Chinese medical system was completed in the first century. For thousands of years the Chinese have observed life processes and relationships between man and nature, the human body and the environment. From this observation and practice, many great medical classics were written, edited, and compiled. To share this vast and rich heritage of Chinese medical art, I wrote (in English) *Chinese Herb Medicine and Therapy, The Way to Good Health with Chinese Herbs,* and a number of articles, books, and monograph series.

John August Rau has attended herb classes taught by myself and M.M. Van Benschoten at OHAI. His enthusiasm and hard work led to the creation of this book, containing our lectures and research and intended as an addition to *Commonly Used Chinese Herb Formulas.* Although this book centers on the treatment of some complicated diseases, further study necessitates extensive reading of the original texts, such as *Huang ti nei ching* (The Yellow Emperor's Classic of Internal Medicine), *Shang han lun* (Treatise on Febrile Diseases), *Shen nung pen ts'ao ching* (The Book on Herbs by Shen Nung), *Chin kuei yao lueh* (Prescriptions from the Golden Chamber), *Mai ching* (Pulse Classic), *Wen ping lun* (Treatise on Epidemic Disease), and *Chu ping yuan ho chung lun* (General Treatise on the Etiology and Symptomatology of Disease), which will come out shortly in English.

Index of Differentiation for Commonly Used Chinese Herb Formulas, which covers a wide range of herbal formulas, deals with differentiation of Chinese herbal medicine, principles of treatment, and the selection of the most appropriate formula for a specific disease. Comprehensive and unique, this book is a must for those who wish to further understand the art of Chinese medicine.

I am indebted to Miss Wang Shu-kuei and Mr. M.M. Van Benschoten for their joint effort in proofreading that has made the publication of this book possible.

Hong-yen Hsu, Ph.D.
President
Oriental Healing Arts Institute

August 1983

Acknowledgements and Introduction

It has been said that, traditionally, one would study the classic texts two years prior to apprenticing ten years under a Master Herbalist before one was competant to prescribe on one's own. In our time, with the pharmacists' role of herbal preparation taken over by firms such as Sun-Ten Pharmaceutical, new practitioners are entrusted with patient care after an institutionalized training of three to four years in East-West therapeutics. In addition, it is hoped that established Western clinicians in the future will find Eastern herbal therapeutics appropriate in clinical situations unresponsive to Western methods, or as an adjunct to Western pharmacology.

From a practical point of view, the utilization problem is an information processing problem. Despite empirically documented resources from many generations of Oriental practice, very little has been translated into English.

Dr. Hong-yen Hsu, founder of the Brion Research Institute, has been a foremost compiler and publisher of Chinese herbal therapeutics. M. M. Van Benschoten aided Dr. Hsu in the English translation of lecture material presented at the Oriental Healing Arts Institute, Los Angeles during 1982-1983. M. M. Van Benschoten's extensive background in Western natural therapeutics and superlative communication skills, made this lecture series a landmark event. It is from these materials that this compendium was compiled.

The core text for syndrome conformations was Dr. Hsu's book, *Commonly Used Chinese Herb Formulas.*

The usual method of classification of Chinese herbal formulations by therapeutic method is difficult for the new practitioner not already skilled in the indications of each formula to use. *Commonly Used Chinese Herb Formulas* is organized by therapeutic method. It is the intention with this compendium to provide an index of differentiation starting from a Western symptom, sign or chief complaint, and through a process of information selection derive the appropriate formulation that most matches the clinical syndrome conformation, as described in detail in Dr. Hsu's book, *Commonly Used Chinese Herb Formulas.*

The Index is divided into two sections: Western Syndromes and Traditional Chinese Medicine Syndromes. All pages, with a few exceptions noted, refer to *Commonly Used Chinese Herb Formulas* by Hsu (or on exception noted, *Natural Healing with Chinese Herbs,* Hsu, ed.).

An asterisk (*) by a formula page number indicates that this formula is routinely stocked by Sun-Ten Pharmaceutical/Brion Corporation, Hawaiian Gardens, California.

It is with great appreciation that I wish to acknowledge the insight and generosity of Hong-yen Hsu and M. M. Van Benschoten, as well as Douglas Easer and the staff of the Oriental Healing Arts Institute, Los Angeles for making possible the perpetuation of the wisdom and experience of generations of Chinese therapeutics within a Western context.

John August Rau, D.D.S.
May 1983

Index of Differentiations in *Commonly Used Herb Formulations,* Hsu

A

* pt: patient w̅: with Tx: treatment

– C –

– D –

– E –

– F –

– G –

– H –

– I –

– L –

* esp. : especially

– M –

– N –

– O –

– P –

– R –

– S –

– T –

– U –

– V –

– W –

– X –

– Y –

Characteristics of Herbs

Floating Drugs –	**Flowers & Leaves**	disperse surface accumulations remove wind; induce sweating warm inside YANG
Sinking Drugs –	**Seeds, Fruits, Minerals, Roots**	concentrate interior fluid and energy YIN

Cooking in wine – enhances the floating nature
Baking in salt – enhances the sinking nature

Cooling –	watery fruits, vegetables melons, sprouts, bamboo, pumpkin, eggplant, cucumber	chrysanthemum/lonicera
Cold –	gypsum	
Warm –	fresh ginger	perilla/peony
Hot –	flesh foods, wine	dry ginger, aconite
Neutral (Bing) –		hoelen, ginseng, codonopsis
Cold Drugs –	cleansing heat, fire, toxicity	
Warm Drugs –	supplementing GI, yang; disperse cold	evodia, zanthoxylum dry ginger, cinnamon, aconite

Yang – pungent, sweet, neutral (*tan*)

Yin – salty, bitter, sour

Pungent – dispersing, sweating; increase *qi* circulation

Sweet – nourish & supplement spleen/stomach

Neutral – diuretic

Bitter – purge/clear fire: dry moisture: aid defecation

Sour – astringent – arrest sweating
arrest diarrhea
arrest expectoration

Aromatic – remove stagnant blood; normalize circulation (*qi*); resuscitate (stroke)

supplement blood
qi
yang
yin

tang-kuei

Herbs to Remove Wind
cinnamon
pueraria
mahuang
siler

Herbs to Remove Moisture
atractylodes
hoelen
stephania
astragalus

Herbs to Remove Stagnant Blood
persica
moutan

Herbs to Supplement Blood
cnidium
tang-kuei

Herbs for Pain
peony
licorice
aconite

Herbs to Supplement Protein
ginseng
dioscorea
tang-shen (codonopsis)

edema/infection/impotence

astragalus
hoelen
soy bean
human placenta

Herbs to Supplement Fatty Acids
skin/hormonal

hide gelatin
lamb
sesame
cannabis seeds
soybean
ginseng

Herbs to Supplement Glucose/Carbohydrate
fatigue

maltose
rehmannia
gastrodia

Herbs with Vitamin A
shao yang anorexia

chicken liver
lotus seed
bat dung
bupleurum
scute
lycium

Herbs with Vitamin B_1
muscular weakness/neuritis

rice sprouts
mume prunes
evodia
crataegus
schizandra
coix
euryale

Herbs with Vitamin B_2
cheilitis, bloodshot eyes, skin

chicken gizzard
schizandra (lung)
lycium (eye)

Herbs with Vitamin B_{12}
beriberi/pernicious anemia/mental acuity

tang-kuei
cnidium
deer horn
tortoise shell
hide gelatin
bupleurum
scute

Herbs with Vitamin C
- citrus peel
- cornus

Herbs with Vitamin D
- mushrooms

Herbs with Vitamin E — arteriosclerosis, muscle atropy, RBC fragility
- atractylodes
- eucommia (sexual)
- artemisia
- cuscuta (sexual)

Herbs with Vitamin K
- pseudoginseng (*tien chi*)
- bletilla
- segetum

Section I
Indication/Differentiation Index by Western Syndrome

ANEMIA
(*Xue Xu*)

Heart/Spleen Yin *Xu*

TX: Supplement *qi*; nourish *ying*	yellowish, dry skin wrinkled palpitations; exhaustion insomnia; many dreams anorexia Tongue – thin pale Pulse – very weak
* p. 433 Tang-kuei Four Combination (*Szu-wu-tang*)	for simple anemia, gynecologic disorders
* p. 239 Ginseng Nutritive Combination (*Jen-sheng-yang-yung-tang*)	severe *qi* deficiency nightsweats
* p. 291 Minor Cinnamon & Peony Comb.* (*Hsiao-chien-chung-tang*)	children
* p. 264 Major Four Herb Combination (*Szu-chun-tzu-tang*)	gastrointestinal weakness (*qi* tonic)
* p. 248 Tang-kuei & Ginseng 8 Comb. (*Pa-chen-tang*)	*qi* and blood deficiency
* p. 425 Ginseng & Longan Combination (*Kuei-pi-tang*)	poor memory; palpitations

Spleen Yang Deficiency

* p. 295 Ginseng & Ginger Combination (*Jen-sheng-tang*) plus ½ gm aconite if severe	pale, exhausted cold limbs; fears cold anorexia loose stools T* – thin; greasy P* – soft; weak
* p. 255 Ginseng & Astragalus Comb. (*Pu-chung-i-chi-tang*) may increase astragalus *tang-kuei*	severe weakness, gastrointestinal dysfunction, rectal or uterine prolapse
p. 262 Ginseng & Tang-kuei 10 Comb. (*Shih-chuan-ta-pu-tang*)	severe post surgical or convalescent anemia

* Comb.: Combination T : Tongue P : Pulse

Worm Accumulation Anemia

p. 569 Mume Formula
(*Wu-mei-wan*)

yellowish face
edema
anorexia; or excessive appetite
abdominal discomfort

Kidney Yang *Xu*

* p. 250 Rehmannia Eight Formula
(*Pa-wei-ti-huang-wan*)

Note: if sp* *xu* do not give rehmannia: upsets stomach use Major 4 Herb Comb.
or
Eucommia & Rehmannia Formula
(*Yu-kuei-wan*)

processed rehmannia	8 gm
dioscorea	4 gm
tang-kuei	3 gm
lycium	4 gm
deer antler gelatin	4 gm
eucommia	4 gm
cinnamon	2 gm
aconite	2 gm
cornus	3 gm
cuscuta	4 gm

external coldness; exhaustion
aversion to cold
plus low back distress, spontaneous sweating, nocturnal emission impotence/menstrual irregularity
T- thin body; white coat
P- thin; small
P- slippery

* p. 248 Tang-kuei Four plus
Major 4 Herb Comb.
= Tang-kuei & Ginseng Eight

acute anemia; early

* p. 190 Coptis & Rhubarb Comb.
(*San-huang-hsieh-hsin-tang*)

hemorrhage anemia of upper heater
epistaxis
hematemesis (bright red)
also non-responsive
'last resort'
menstrual bleeding

* p. 576 Tang-kuei & Gelatin Comb.
(*Chiung-kuei-chiao-ai-tang*)

hemorrhage anemia of lower heater
menstrual
hemorrhoid (dark red)

* p. 439 Tang-kuei & Gardenia Comb.
(*Wen-ching-yin*)

if dry skin, hot flashes or flushed face

---

* sp : spleen

Page	Formula	Indication
* p. 175	Coptis & Scute Combination (*Huang-lien-chieh-tu-tang*)	hemorrhage anemia of middle heater GI ulcer strong patient
* p. 295	Ginseng & Ginger Combination (*Jen-sheng-tang*)	if weak patient w̄ chills
* p. 493	Atractylodes & Hoelen Comb. (*Ling-kuei-chu-kan-tang*)	if irregular urination dizziness/palpitations
p. 427	Tang-kuei & Atractylodes Comb. (*Lien-chu-yin*)	anemia w̄ menstrual irregularity dry skin
* p. 311	G.L. & Aconite with Ginseng Comb. (*Szu-ni-chia-jen-sheng-tang*) or Fu-lung-kan Combination	severe acute hemorrhage anemia (post-surgery anemia) cold extremities dry heaves/palpitations pale P- fast but imperceptible
	Li-ban-wan *Atractylodes lancea* 8 gm citrus peel 8 gm magnolia bark 8 gm jujube 8 gm *shen-chu* 8 gm licorice 5 gm burned copper sulfate 4 gm (until black)	anemia due to worms make aduki-sized pills 30 pills/day
* p. 425	Ginseng & Longan Combination (*Kuei-pi-tang*)	idiopathic anemia and leukemia
* p. 264	Major Four Herb Combination (*Szu-chun-tzu-tang*)	stomach ulceration/cancer anemia w̄ *qi xu*
* p. 432	Tang-kuei Four Combination (*Szu-wu-tang*) or	anemia due to hemorrhage
* p. 248	Tang-kuei & Ginseng 8 Comb. (*Pa-chen-tang*)	
p. 427	Tang-kuei & Atractylodes (*Lien-chu-yin*)	anemia with "water toxicity" (palpitations, dizziness, tinnitis, headache w̄ edema)
* p. 262	Ginseng & Tang-kuei 10 Comb. (*Shih-chuan-ta-pu-tang*)	anemia after long illness esp. uterine cancer, TB of bones dry skin

* p. 585	Tang-kuei & Peony Comb. (*Tang-kuei-shao-yao-san*)	anemia, postpartum
* p. 351	Cinnamon & Dragon Bone Comb. (*Kuei-chih-chia-lung-ku-mu-li-tang*)	anemia in children
* p. 425	Ginseng & Longan Comb. (*Kuei-pi-tang*)	anemia of chronic hemorrhage peptic ulcer hemorrhoids

ASTHMA

* p. 407	*Ting-chuan-tang* (Mahuang & Gingko Combination) "soothing asthma tea"	asthmatic cough w̄ mucus; strong no sweating (internal heat)
* p. 199	*Tzu-yin-chiang-huo-tang* (Phellodendron Combination) "nourish yin; suppress fire"	DRY asthmatic cough; TB (dry rales) constipation (yin *xu* heat) no sweating (except night)
* p. 538	*Mai-men-tung-yin-tzu* (Ophiopogon & Trichosanthes)	chronic dry cough, thirst w̄ general weakness; dry skin-coarse; anemia
* p. 91 * p. 395	Minor Bupleurum Formula Pinellia & Magnolia Comb. 50:50	PEDIATRIC cough/asthma
* p. 395	Pinellia & Magnolia Combination (*Pan-hsia-hou-pu-tang*)	asthma attack due to emotional stress

WIND-CHILL STRONG ASTHMA

* p. 43	*Hsiao-ching-lung-tang* (Minor Blue Dragon Comb.)	thin clear sputum; stagnant water stomach, surface fever
* p. 47	*Hua-kai-san* (Mahuang & Morus Comb.)	long term; children GI distress, poor appetite

DRY HEAT STRONG ASTHMA

* p. 78	*Sang-chu-yin* (Morus & Chrysanthemum)	mild
* p. 537	*Mai-men-tung-tang* (Ophiopogon Comb.)	severe, dry cough
* p. 173	*Hsieh-pai-san*	(most) severe:

(Morus & Lycium Comb.)	add trichosanthes root adenophora platycodon ophiopogon
p. 401 *Wu-hu-erh-chen-tang* (Gypsum, Citrus, & Pinellia Combination)	LONG TERM ADMINISTRATION (Similar to Mahuang & Apricot)

LUNG WEAKNESS

p. 553 *Kua-lou-chih-shih-tang* (Trichosanthes & Chih-shih)	chest full/pain; thick sputum dry mouth, dark urine
* p. 401 *Shen-mi-tang* (Mahuang & Magnolia Comb.)	more severe; abdominal weakness melancholia, neurosis
p. 258 *Pu-fei-ah-chiao-tang* (Gelatin & Aristolochia Comb.) equal to Ophiopogon Comb.	severe kidney-lung weakness dry throat; hemoptysis; red tongue no coat

KIDNEY WEAKNESS

* p. 250 *Pa-wei-ti-huang-wan* (Rehmannia 8 Formula)	kidney yang *xu*
* p. 245 *Liu-wei-ti-huang-wan* (Rehmannia 6 Formula)	kidney yin *xu*
p. 226 Rehmannia & Schizandra = Rehmannia 7 (*Chi-wei-tu-chi-wan*) Rehmannia 6 plus schizandra	combined lu★/ki★ weakness severe cough w sputum in weak pt also sore throat, hoarseness

Asthma differential: p. 401 & 554

BLADDER INFECTIONS

DAMP HEAT

* p. 181 Gentiana Combination (*Lung-tan-hsieh-kan-tang*)	strong patient, heat sensations in genitals
* p. 502 Dianthus Formula (*Pa-cheng-san*)	more severe; strong patient fever, constipation gonorrhealike dripping urination

★ lu : lung ki : kidney

* p. 472	Polyporus Combination (*Chu-ling-tang*)	blood in urine; severe urinary pain ki yang *xu* w̄ edema, diarrhea
* p. 250	Rehmannia 8 Formula (*Pa-wei-ti-huang-wan*)	extreme weakness, senility; cystitis bladder atrophy (cystatrophy) prostate problems not if GI weakness, diarrhea

BREAST CANCER

* p. 632	Lithospermum & Oyster Shell (*Tzu-ken-mu-li-tang*)	lymphadenoma; anemia, weak malignant skin disorders
* p. 402	Tang-kuei 16 Herb Combination (*Shih-liu-wei-liu-chi-yin*)	cervical lymphadenopathy, goiter fibrocystic disease
* p. 617	W. T. T. C. (*Lo-shih-shu*) plus	to prevent post-surgical metasteses
* p. 242	Major Six Herb Combination (*Liu-chun-tzu-tang*)	

CARDIAC DISTRESS

ANGINA/PALPITATIONS

p. 529	Baked Licorice Combination (*Chih-kan-tsao-tang*) 6 gm daily, 1-3 years	palpitation from hyperthyroid goiter; exopthalmic (*yin xu* heat) tachycardia, irregular thin; nervousness spontaneous sweating abdom* /umbilical palpitation fragile hair
p. 87	Bupleurum & Peony Comb. (*Chia-wei-hsiao-yao-san*)	goiter in females w̄ menstrual irregularity nervousness
p. 103	Pinellia & Licorice Comb. (*Kan-tsao-hsieh-hsin-tang*)	goiter w̄ diarrhea
p. 500	Stephania & Ginseng Comb. (*Mu-fang-chi-tang*)	palpitation from valvular disease edema, dyspnea pale, anemic

* abdom : abdominal

		cough w̄ sputum oliguria
p. 340	Bupleurum & Dragon Bone Comb. (*Chai-hu-chia-lung-ku-mu-li-tang*)	palpitation, neurotic dyspnea constipation easily frightened
p. 85	Bupleurum, Cinnamon, & Dry Ginger (*Chai-hu-kuei-chih-kan-chiang-tang*)	if weak pt
p. 395	Pinellia & Magnolia Comb. (*Pan-hsia-hou-pu-tang*)	palpitation, hysteric (intermittent but severe) paroxysmal atrial tachycardia anxious, fearful use scalp pt "thoracic cavity"
p. 495	Hoelen, Licorice, & Jujube Comb. (*Ling-kuei-kan-tsao-tang*) cinnamon 4 gm licorice 2 gm hoelen 6 gm jujube 4 gm	if *qi* rising/flush dizziness, headache uterine spasm if anemia, also: *Szu-wu-tang*

ANGINA/PALPITATIONS

p. 500	Stephania & Ginseng Comb. (*Mu-fang-chi-tang*)	palpitation w̄ cardiac asthma dyspnea w̄ edema flushing; thirst
p. 397	Areca & Evodia Combination (*Pien-chih-hsin-chi-yin*)	if stiff shoulders; hepatomegaly/angina
p. 495	Hoelen, Licorice, & Jujube Comb. (*Ling-kuei-kan-tsao-tang*)	if flushing w̄ vertigo
p. 340	Bupleurum & Dragon Bone Combination	cardiac neurosis paroxysmal atrial tachycardia (functional heart disease) strong pt chest distress constipation insomnia
p. 351	Cinnamon & Dragon Bone	if slightly weak
p. 480	Hoelen, Apricot, & Licorice (*Fu-ling-hsing-jen-kan-tsao-tang*) hoelen 6 gm apricot seed 4 gm licorice 1 gm	if weak, severe chest pain

CIRCULATORY DISORDERS

CARDIAC

p. 340	Bupleurum & Dragon Bone (*Chai-hu-chia-lung-ku-mu-li-tang*)	mild chest distress hypertension dyspnea emotional instability nervousness, insomnia
(p. 82)*	Siler and Platycodon Formula (*Fang-feng-tung-sheng-san*)	hypertension in obese w̄ constipation
p. 493	Hoelen & Atractylodes (*Ling-kuei-chu-kan-tang*)	dizziness, esp. elderly "water toxin in head" palpitations motion sickness valvular heart disease/edema hysteric neurasthenia
p. 500	Stephania & Ginseng Comb. (*Mu-fang-chi-tang*)	valvular heart disease/edema asthmatic flushing up thirst; oliguria hardness below heart
p. 349	Licorice Combination (*Kan-tsao-tang*) = Licorice 8 gm/dose	goiter; sore throat, visceral spasm dry cough-bronchiospasm
p. 397	Areca & Evodia Combination (*Pien-chih-hsin-chi-yin*)	if Stephania & Ginseng ineffective angina pectoris shoulder/back stiffness

HYPERTENSION/ARTERIOSCLEROSIS

p. 128	Major Bupleurum Combination (*Ta-chai-hu-tang*)	hypertension in strong pt chest distress constipation
p. 190	Coptis & Rhubarb Comb. (*San-huang-hsieh-hsin-tang*)	hypertension in strong pt severe facial flushing (heat) easily angers insomnia constipation
p. 175	Coptis & Scute Combination (*Huang-lien-chieh-tu-tang*)	if no constipation and flushed
p. 340	Bupleurum & Dragon Bone (*Chai-hu-chia-lung-ku-mu-li-tang*)	hypertension in WEAK pt with nervousness

p. 250	Rehmannia 8 Formula (*Pa-wei-ti-huang-wan*)	hypertension in weak, elderly low back pain weak lower extremities
p. 493	Hoelen & Atractylodes Comb. (*Ling-kuei-chu-kan-tang*)	hypertension w̄ vertigo, dyspnea asthmatic headache
p. 386	Gambir Formula (*Tou-teng-san*)	hypertension w̄ MORNING headache tinnitus
p. 415	Tang-kuei & Gambir Comb. (*Chi-wu-chiang-hsia-tang*)	hypertension in WEAK pt heavy head w̄ tinnitis flushing up nephritis
p. 448	Mahuang & Ginseng Combination (*Hsu-ming-tang*)	POST-STROKE preventive

COMMON COLD
Gan Mau

* p. 76	Mahuang Combination (*Ma-huang-tang*)	strong pt; surface fever **no sweating**; general ache
* p. 51	Pueraria Combination (*Ko-ken-tang*)	strong pt; **stiff neck, back** not as severe general ache **no sweating**; possible diarrhea
* p. 108	Peony & Licorice Combination (*Shao-yao-kan-tsao-tang*)	add if acute muscle pain/ spasm use *Ko-ken-tang* if mahuang upsets stomach
* p. 63	Cinnamon Combination (*Kuei-chih-tang*)	weak pt; **sweating**; chills/fever general ache, dry heaves abdominal pain
* p. 43	Minor Blue Dragon Combination (*Hsiao-ching-lung-tang*)	strong pt; water toxin in stomach wind-cold phobia; vertigo asthmatic cough/breathing diarrhea; **watery secretions** rhinitis conjunctivitis

* p. 81	Major Blue Dragon Combination (*Ta-ching-lung-tang*)	strong pt; severe internal fever no sweating, irritable thirst/edema (more severe water accumulation)
p. 62	Cinnamon & Mahuang Comb. (*Kuei-chih-ma-huang-ko-pan-tang*)	external heat: **itching**, flush no sweating, less chill/pain no constipation
p. 526	Mahuang & Gypsum Com. (*Yueh-pi-tang*) (1 part) plus	weak pt; extreme thirst, edema spont. **sweating**, oliguria asthmatic cough
* p. 63	Cinnamon Combination (2 parts) (*Kuei-chih-tang*)	or Major Blue Dragon: Cinnamon 1 : 2
* p. 72	Mahuang & Asarum Combination (*Ma-huang-fu-tzu-hsi-hsin-tang*)	weak pt; pale, chills, extreme fatigue, general ache, watery sputum/cough, freq, profuse urination

WIND-COLD
winter, spring

* p. 41	Cyperus & Perilla Formula (*Hsiang-su-san*) weak pt w̄ GI distress nausea, heavy head stagnant food (also for fish poisoning) stiff shoulders	no sweating no thirst clear rhinitis or stuffed/sneezing chill/fever/general ache 3-7 day duration external cold P – tense, tight but not slow T – white fur
* p. 609	Schizonepeta & Siler Formula (*Ching-fang-pai-tu-san*)	severe nasal/sinus congestion chill/fever, muscle spasm esp. if suppurative skin
* p. 81	Major Blue Dragon Combination (*Ta-ching-lung-tang*)	thirst; edema; internal fever strong pt.

WIND-HEAT

* p. 78	Morus & Chrysanthemum Comb. (*Sang-chu-yin*)	sweating thirst, dry mouth, sore throat nosebleed if severe heat red eyes P–floating & fast T–red w̄ white coat

Page	Formula	Indication
* p. 83	Lonicera & Forsythia Formula (*Yin-chiao-san*)	less throat soreness, more irritability, tonsillitis initial measles/mumps
p. 38	Chianghuo Combination (*Chiu-wei-chiang-huo-tang*) or *Chiang-huo-ching-su-tang* *chianghuo* 3 gm *tu-huo* 3 gm *kao-pen* 1.5 gm siler 1.5 gm baked licorice 1.5 gm (honey fried) cnidium 1.5 gm vitex 0.9 gm	WIND-DAMP: heavy head/cold weak extremities bone pain (joints) rheumatic **no thirst**, mild fever P- floating & soft T- thick white coat
p. 221	Elsholtzia Combination (*Hsiang-ju-yin*)	RETAINED SUMMER HEAT fever, thirst, chest distress continuous sweating reddish urine/edema P- slippery T- thick yellow
p. 218	Astragalus & Atractylodes Comb. (*Ching-shu-i-chi-tang*) heatstroke	
* p. 35	Bupleurum & Pueraria Comb. (*Chai-ko-chieh-chi-tang*)	DAMP-HEAT w̄ very high fever, thirst, epistaxis, general ache no sweating, pneumonia
* p. 58	Minor Pueraria Combination (*Hsiao-ko-ken-tang*) = Cinnamon & Pueraria Comb.	WIND-COLD w̄ stiff neck but in weak pt w̄ sweating
* p. 63	Cinnamon Combination (*Kuei-chih-tang*)	WIND-COLD in weak pt; sweating but no stiffneck
* p. 79	Mahuang & Cimicifuga Comb. (*Shih-shen-tang*)	fever but severe chills stuffy nose, chest distress no sweating; hoarse cough
p. 594	Cimicifuga & Pueraria Comb. (*Sheng-ma-ko-ken-tang*)	**dry nose,** body aches (including eyes) no sweating, insomnia, thirst
* p. 37	Pueraria Nasal Combination (*Ching-pi-tang*)	rhinitis, general fatigue, sore throat, also stuffy nose stiff neck, shoulders
* p. 40	Cnidium & Tea Formula (*Chuan-chiung-cha-tiao-san*)	WIND-COLD w̄ vertigo, headache, congestion
* p. 46	Apricot Seed & Perilla Formula (*Hsing-su-san*)	WIND-COLD w̄ stuffy nose gastrointestinal distress

p. 54	Cinnamon, Magnolia, & Apricot Seed (*Kuei-chih-chia-hou-pu-hsing-jen-tang*)	WIND-COLD w̄ cough, bronchitis congestion
* p. 47	Mahuang & Morus Formula (*Hua-kai-san*)	WIND-COLD asthmatic wheezing esp. children
* p. 55	Cinnamon & Astragalus Comb. (*Kuei-chih-chia-huang-chi-tang*) or	WIND-COLD in WEAK pt; cold limbs
* p. 63	Cinnamon Combination (*Kuei-chih-tang*)	weak pt/chills severe
* p. 72	Mahuang & Asarum Comb. (*Ma-huang-fu-tzu-hsi-hsin-tang*)	WIND-COLD in very weak; **elderly** with cold limbs
p. 68	Mahuang & Apricot Seed Comb. (*Ma- hsing-kan-shih-tang*)	**WIND-HEAT** in weak pt; GI distress
* p. 48	Ginseng & Mentha Formula (*Jen-sheng-pai-tu-san*) or	DAMP-HEAT, stuffy nose, general rheumatic ache, stiff neck no sweating congestion
* p. 50	Pueraria & Magnolia Comb. (*Ko-ken-chia-hsin-i-chuan-chiung*)	

CONSTIPATION

Constipation due to internal heat

p. 141	Minor Rhubarb Combination (*Hsiao-cheng-chi-tang*)	w̄ sweating/HICCOUGHS
p. 145	Major Rhubarb Combination (*Ta-cheng-chi-tang*)	more severe heat w̄ extreme thirst, delirium, dyspnea spont. sweat/black dry fur
p. 154	Rhubarb & Mirabilitum Comb. (*Tiao-wei-cheng-chi-tang*)	irritable, no chill; no spont. sweating
**p. 435	Persica & Rhubarb Combination (*Tao-ho-cheng-chi-tang*)	general buring sensation dysmenorrhea hypersensitivity/hysteria
p. 535	Apricot Seed & Linum Formula (*Ma-tzu-jen-wan*)	weak, elderly dry skin, freq.* urination

* freq. : frequent

	Formula	Dose	Indication
			Constipation due to internal cold
p. 150	Rhubarb & Aconite Combination (*Ta-huang-fu-tzu-tang*)		unilateral hypochondrial pain/spasm relieved by warmth
	rhubarb	1 gm	pale lips/mouth
	asarum	2 gm	clear urine
	aconite	½-1 gm	P – sinking/slow
	or		T – fur white
	Pinellia and Sulfur Formula (*Pan-liu-wan*)		
	pinellia	15 gm	
	sulfur	10 gm	sulfur produces foul gas for weeks
	honey to make pills	3-6 gm ea (per dose)	
			Constipation due to stagnant *qi*
* p. 405	Perilla Fruit Combination (*Su-tzu-chiang-chi-tang*)		acid regurgitation/neurosis heart/abdominal discomfort
	or		tight/full rectus abdom.
	Liu-ma-yin		weak
	clove	2 gm	P- tight, big
	saussurea	2 gm	T- body narrow w̅ pointed tip
	areca	2 gm	cold feet
	lindera	2 gm	
	poncirus	2 gm	
	rhubarb	2 gm	
**p. 535	Apricot Seed & Linum Formula (*Ma-tzu-jen-wan*)		weak stomach/nausea/thirst dizziness/thin physique
	freq.urination		pale lips/sweating
	floating pulse		weakness after defecation
	or		dypsnea
**p. 533	Linum & Rhubarb Combination (*Jun-chang-tang*)		dry skin, mouth
	elderly		
	rabbitlike, dry feces		
			WIND Constipation
p. 141/145	Major/Minor Rhubarb Comb.		strong pt post-stroke
	or		catches cold easily
p. 154	Rhubarb & Mirabilitum Comb.		dizziness/hot w̅ fever heat in stomach/abdom fullness
			Generally Used Formulas
**p. 128	Major Bupleurum Combination		Strong pt w̅ chest distress

	(*Ta-chai-hu-tang*)	gallbladder disease hypertension obesity
**p. 119	Siler & Platycodon Formula (*Fang-feng-tung-sheng-san*)	obesity & chronic constipation w̄ flushing up
p. 145	Major Rhubarb Combination (*Ta-cheng-chi-tang*)	tight abdomen/tight umbilicus
**p. 190	Coptis & Rhubarb Combination (*San-huang-hsieh-hsin-tang*)	red faced/irritable/anxious insomnia infra cardiac discomfort
**p. 533	Linum & Rhubarb Combination (*Jun-chang-tang*)	dry mucous membranes chronic geriatric constipation
* p. 535	Apricot Seed & Linum Formula	post illness constipation w̄ weakness
* p. 315	Major Zanthoxylum Combination (*Ta-chien-chung-tang*) or	tenesemus w̄ straining at stool or where purgatives produce abdominal pain
* p. 60	Cinnamon & Peony Comb. plus ginseng 2 gm zanthoxylum 2 gm	esp. w̄ gas & abdominal weak

Four *Cheng-Chi* Formulas — strong patient: large, long stools; tenesemus/strain

p. 145	Major Rhubarb Combination (*Ta-cheng-chi-tang*)	acute febrile disease severe diarrhea/strong pt hypertension **constipation of pregnancy**
* p. 141	Minor Rhubarb Combination (*Hsiao-cheng-chi-tang*)	less severe
p. 154	Rhubarb & Mirabilitum Comb. (*Tiao-wei-cheng-chi-tang*)	slightly weak pt
* p. 435	Persica & Rhubarb Combination (*Tao-ho-cheng-chi-tang*)	*xue yu* w̄ cramping (dysmenorrhea) flushing/hypertension/hysteria general burning sensation tendency to obesity
p. 379	Magnolia Three Combination (*Hou-po-san-wu-tang*) magnolia bark 8 gm	constipation (habitual) with **respiratory** obstruction asthma

	Formula	Indication
	rhubarb 4 gm *chih-shih* 3.5 gm	hypertension
* p. 519	Capillaris Combination (*Yin-chen-hao-tang*)	w̄ jaundice & thirst strong yellow urine
* p. 128	Major Bupleurum Combination (*Ta-chai-hu-tang*) or	strong conformation red face stiff shoulders
* p. 190	Coptis & Rhubarb Combination (*San-huang-hsieh-hsin-tang*)	
p. 152	Rhubarb & Licorice Combination (*Ta-huang-kan-tsao-tang*) rhubarb 4 gm licorice 1 gm	chronic constipation 3 gm/day
* p. 535	Apricot Seed & Linum Formula (*Ma-tzu-jen-wan*) or	weak patient rabbit-pellet stools fear of cold profuse urination dry skin
* p. 533	Linum & Rhubarb Combination (*Jun-chang-tang*)	
* p. 124	Cinnamon & Peony Comb. plus rhubarb	*tai* yin stage weak, cold post surgical constipation
p. 150	Rhubarb & Aconite Combination	*tai* yin strong, cold legs geriatric constipation
* p. 242	Major Six Herb Combination (*Liu-chun-tzu-tang*) followed by	weak, nervous pt stiff shoulders/flushing hot/cold sensation in back
* p. 87	Bupleurum & Peony Formula (*Chia-wei-hsiao-yao-san*)	post-hysterectomy digestive disorder constipation
* p. 291	Minor Cinnamon & Peony Comb. (*Hsiao-chien-chung-tang*)	*tai* yin weak; easily fatigued soft abdomen-navel but tight rectus abdominis

COUGH

	Formula	Indication
* p. 169	*Ching-yen-li-ke-tang* (Arctium Combination) "cleanse throat, smooth diaphragm tea"	SORE THROAT, chest distress tonsillitis, constipation

Exogenous Infection Cough

	Formula	Differentiation
* p. 43	*Hsiao-ching-lung-tang* (Minor Blue Dragon Comb.)	chill
p. 546	*Chih-sou-san* (Platycodon & Schizonepeta) "crowing (whooping) cough"	chill Whooping Cough/laryngitis/ headache, less sputum
* p. 41	*Hsiang-su-san* (Cyperus & Perilla Formula)	chill, cough, & food stagnation heavy head abdominal pain of emotional origin (if Cinnamon Combination or *Ko-ken-tang* (Pueraria Combination) ineffective)
* p. 78	*Sang-chu-yin* (Morus & Chrysanthemum)	HEAT Cough, thick sticky phlegm
* p. 175	*Huang-lien-chieh-tu-tang* (Coptis & Scute Combination)	HEAT Cough (severe internal heat)
* p. 548	*Ching-fei-tang* (Platycodon & Fritillaria Comb.) "Cleanse Lung Tea"	HEAT Cough, milder (combine w̄ above) thick sputum
* p. 537	*Mai-men-tung-tang* (Ophiopogon Combination)	DRY cough, sore throat combine w̄ above in severe case

Acute Cough

	Formula	Differentiation
* p. 43	*Hsiao-ching-lung-tang* (Minor Blue Dragon Comb.)	DRY cough or clear secretions *tai* yang- clear nasal strong, no sweating
p. 68	*Ma-hsing-kan-shih-tang* (Mahuang & Apricot Comb.)	severe cough w̄ fever (mild) Children spontaneous sweating, thirst
* p. 81	*Ta-ching-lung-tang* (Major Blue Dragon Comb.)	severe cough; **no sweating**; strong thirst (internal heat); edema/ascites *tai* yang fever, chills, ache ANXIETY, IRRITABILITY severe

Chronic Cough

	Formula	Differentiation
* p. 548	*Ching-fei-tang* (Platycodon & Fritillaria Comb.) "cleansing lung tea"	CHRONIC COUGH - "Smoker's cough" thick yellow phlegm

Page	Formula	Indications
* p. 537	*Mai-men-tung-tang* (Ophiopogon Combination)	DRY COUGH, sore throat, hoarseness
* p. 72	*Ma-huang-fu-tzu-hsi-hsin-tang* (Mahuang & Asarum Combination)	yang *xu* chronic cough; coldness weak, elderly; stiffness, thin clear expectoration
* p. 556	*Ling-kan-chiang-wei-hsin-hsia-jen-tang* (Hoelen & Schizandra Combination)	chronic yang *xu* emphysema elderly; anemic, palpitations pulmonary edema
* p. 47	*Hua-kai-san* (Mahuang & Morus Comb.)	cough/chest distress $\overline{w}$ nasal congest and GI weakness $\overline{w}$ poor appetite
p. 553	*Kua-lou-chih-shih-tang* (Trichosanthes & Chih-shih Comb.)	SMOKER'S cough with constipation
p. 253	*Pai-ho-ku-chin-tang* (Lily Combination)	TB, kidney weakness; hemoptysis
p. 220	*Chu-yeh-shih-kao-tang* (Bamboo Leaves & Gypsum Combination)	TB, weakness severe thirst, night sweats dry skin, constipation severe internal heat-insomnia nightmares P – weak but rapid

Cough due to internal injury

Page	Formula	Indications
**p. 199	*Tzu-yin-chiang-huo-tang* (Phellodendron Combination)	yin *xu* heat, no sweating dry mouth, constipation
p. 189	*Pu-chi-hsiao-tu-yin* (Scute & Cimicifuga Comb.)	yin *xu* heat throat pain, swelling TB, mumps
* p. 242	*Liu-chun-tzu-tang* (Major Six Herb Comb.) plus dry ginger schizandra	yang *xu*, severe; sputum GI weakness
* p. 264	*Szu-chun-tzu-tang* (Major 4 Herb Comb.)	yang *xu*, milder; dry mouth
* p. 255	*Pu-chung-i-chi-tang* (Ginseng & Astragalus Comb.)	yang *xu*, fatigue, poor appetite diarrhea after eating weak pt spontaneous sweating
p. 226	Rehmannia & Schizandra Formula = Rehmannia 7	combined lu/ki yang *xu* in weak patient

(*Chi-wei-tu-chi-wan*)
Rehmannia 6 plus schizandra

severe cough w̄ sputum
also sore throat/hoarseness

p.148 Rhubarb & Kan-sui Combination
(*Ta-hsien -hsiung-tang*)
rhubarb 9 gm
mirabilitum 15 gm
Euphorbia kan-sui 1.5 gm

strong pt w̄ damp heat/pain in chest
pulmonary edema
emphysema/pulmonary abscess

p. 142 Minor Trichosanthes Comb.
(*Hsiao-hsien-hsiung-tang*)
coptis 1.5 gm
pinellia 6 gm
trichosanthes seed 3 gm

concentrated sputum/heat in chest
asthmatic breathing
severe chest pain on coughing

or

***p. 543 Bupleurum & Scute Comb.
(*Chai-hsien-tang*)
Diff: Minor Bupleurum
full chest but
no pain
no thick sputum
no difficult expectoration

above w̄
palpitations/dyspnea
bitter taste T- yellow coat
pleurisy
pneumonia/bronchitis
hepatitis
common cold

DIARRHEA

FIVE MOST IMPORTANT FORMULAS:

p. 105 Pinellia Combination
(*Pan-hsia-hsieh-hsin-tang*)

strong pt w̄ acute gastroenteritis

p. 254 Pinellia & Ginseng Six Comb.
(*Pan-hsieh-liu-chun-tzu-tang*)
= Pinellia Comb. + Major Six Comb.

if weaker pt, chronic disorders

p. 123 Pueraria, Coptis, & Scute Comb.
(*Ko-ken-huang-lien-huang-chin-tang*)

if bacterial (damp heat: tenesmus)
fever, sweating
he* fire/shoulder stiff

p. 278 Vitality Combination
(*Chen-wu-tang*)

if extremely weak/chronic w̄/edema
if no effect, use Lotus & Citrus Combination

p. 516 Hoelen Five Herb Formula
(*Wu-ling-san*)

children's stomach flu w̄ thirst
vomiting of fluids

---

* he : heart

Formula	Indication
"SPLEEN" diarrhea (Sp *qi xu*)	
p. 260 Ginseng & Atractylodes Formula (*Sheng-ling-pai-chu-san*)	pale or yellowish complexion/anemic fatigue, anorexia; P- weak
or	
p. 255 Ginseng & Astragalus Comb. (*Pu-chung-i-chi-tang*)	weaker still, spontaneous sweats
"KIDNEY" diarrhea	**Early Morning Diarrhea; Abdominal Pain Reflexed to Lumbar Back**
p. 325 Evodia Combination (*Wu-chu-yu-tang*)	ki yang *xu* w̄ vomiting, headaches nocturnal emissions
or	
p. 266 Dioscorea Combination (*Szu-shen-tang*) "Four Wonders/Spirits Tea" cooked w̄ pig intestines (menudo)	tonic for heart/spleen/kidney esp. if EDEMA
p. 212 Citrus & Crataegus Formula (*Pao-ho-wan*)	Food excess diarrhea B.M. relieves distress stool yellow, mucous foul breath full abdomen, chest
or	
* p. 104 Cardamon Combination (*Liu-ho-tang*)	
* p. 516 Hoelen 5 Herb Formula (*Wu-ling-san*)	Dampness diarrhea watery stools heavy feeling chest/abdomen distress; full, weak irregular urination glassy, wet tongue
or	
* p. 512 Magnolia & Hoelen Comb. (*Wei-ling-tang*)	
or	
* p. 100 Agastache Formula (*Huo-hsiang-cheng-chi-san*)	
* p. 295 Ginseng & Ginger Comb. (*Jen-sheng-tang*)	Cold diarrhea- "duck stools" undigested food mild continuous lower abdominal pain relieved by warmth T – white coat P – slow
* p. 122 Pueraria, Coptis, & Scute Comb. (*Ko-ken-huang-lien-huang-chin-tang*)	Heat diarrhea burning sensation in anus dry mouth/prefers cold drink reddish urine dysuria T – yellow coat P – rapid
or	
Hsiang-lien-wan saussurea 3 gm coptis 12 gm	

Page	Formulation	Amount	Indications
p. 221	Elsholtzia Combination (*Hsiang-ju-yin*) plus coptis	 1.8 gm	Summertime diarrhea–more severe heat, thirst irritable reddish urine spontaneous sweating
			Diarrhea with Borborygmus; Discomfort in heart after defecation
* p. 105	Pinellia Combination (*Pan-hsia-hsieh-hsin-tang*)		poor appetite; dry heaves (if 2-3x/day)
* p. 110	Pinellia & Ginger Comb. (*Sheng-chiang-hsieh-hsin-tang*)		(if foul odor); acid regurgitation
* p. 103	Pinellia & Licorice Comb. (*Kan-tsao-hsieh-hsin-tang*)		(if more than 3x/day, or more acute conditions) dry heaves, dyspnea mental instability (sp/he)
	Sheng-ho-shao-yao-tang peony *tang-kuei* coptis scute rhubarb saussurea cinnamon licorice	 6 gm 3 gm 3 gm 3 gm 2 gm 1 gm 1 gm 1 gm	tenesmus w̅ painful lower abdomen spastic rectus abdominis painful on pressure =bacterial infection T–brown or yellow dry coat P–strong & fast
* p. 278	Vitality Combination (*Chen-wu-tang*)		chronic diarrhea watery after meals but mild abdominal discomfort chill abdomen weak P – weak
p. 461	Atractylodes & Setaria Comb. (*Wei-feng-tang*)		chronic with blood/mucous
* p. 516	Hoelen 5 Herb Formula (*Wu-ling-san*)		diarrhea w̅ thirst irregular urination no tenesmus esp. children summertime flu
* p. 60	Cinnamon & Peony Comb. (*Kuei-chih-chia-shao-yao-tang*) if more severe pain and ½-1 gm rhubarb		if abdominal pain AFTER defecation rectus abdominis tense P- big but weak = mild L.I.* infection
p. 204	Lotus & Citrus Comb. (*Chi-pi-tang*)		chronic intestinal infection

* L.I.: large intestine

Page	Formula	Indication
p. 51	Pueraria Combination (*Ko-ken-tang*)	acute colitis; bacterial dysentery (epidemic childrens diarrhea) fever, chills, abdom pain tenesmus
p. 122	Pueraria, Coptis, & Scute Comb. (*Ko-ken-huang-lien-huang-chin tang*)	children's diarrhea w̄ high fever, convulsions
p. 228	Atractylodes & Pueraria Formula (*Chien-shih-pai-chu-san*)	infantile indigestion; vomiting of milk
p. 60	Cinnamon & Peony Combination (*Kuei-chih-shao-yao-tang*)	acute colitis; dysentery weak pt
		Otsuka Commentary
p. 103	Pinellia & Licorice Comb. (*Kan-tsao-hsieh-hsin-tang*)	diarrhea 1-2x/day w̄ borborygmus hardness below heart pain relieved on defecation yellowish stool
	if worsens use:	
p. 295	Ginseng & Ginger Comb. (*Jen-sheng-tang*) or	severe pain ABOVE umbilicus (diarrhea 2-3x/day)
p. 278	Vitality Combination (*Chen-wu-tang*)	(diarrhea 3+/day)
p. 110	Pinellia & Ginger Comb. (*Sheng-chiang-hsieh-hsin-tang*)	w̄ GAS, undigested food/ mucous dry heaves acid regurgitation
p. 122	Pueraria, Coptis, & Scute Combination	severe abdominal pain w̄ diarrhea strong patient
p. 278	Vitality Combination	weak patient especially colitis pt on corticosteroids
p. 250	Rehmannia Eight Formula (*Pa-wei-ti-huang-wan*) if worsens, use	diabetic or nephrotic diarrhea
p. 516	Hoelen 5 Herb Formula (*Wu-ling-san*)	w̄ vomiting, nausea
* p. 313	Aconite, Ginger, & Licorice Comb. (*Szu-ni-tang*) licorice 3 gm ginger 2 gm aconite ½-1 gm	sudden severe vomiting w̄ diarrhea in weak, debilitated patient chill, cold limbs

	or	
p. 283	Hoelen, G.L. & Aconite Comb. (*Fu-ling-szu-ni-tang*) = *Szu-ni-tang* + ginseng; hoelen	
* p. 117	Bupleurum & Cinnamon (with added peony) (*Chai-hu-kuei-chih-tang*) 2x	emotional or stress induced diarrhea

Diarrhea with Thirst

p. 187	Anemone Comb. (*Pai-tou-weng-tang*)	strong pt
* p. 98	Coptis Combination (*Huang-lien-tang*)	weak pt; infectious heat, tenesmus
* p. 278	Vitality Combination	severe weakness, cold extremities edema
	or	
* p. 313	Aconite & G. L. Comb.	
* p. 516	Hoelen 5 Herb Formula	with dysuria but no tenesmus

Tenesmus with Diarrhea

* p. 128	Major Bupleurum Comb.	with chest distress
* p. 60	Cinnamon & Peony Comb.	weak pt
* p. 278	Vitality Combination	weaker pt
* p. 287	Aconite, Ginseng, & Ginger Comb.	weaker pt
* p. 313	Aconite, Ginger, & Licorice Comb.	weakest pt
* p. 60	Cinnamon & Peony Combination	induced diarrhea/abdominal pain purgative
p. 617	W.T.T.C.	If nothing works, suspect cancer severe continuous diarrhea

DIZZINESS/VERTIGO

p. 493	Atractylodes & Hoelen Comb. (*Ling-kuei-chu-kan-tang*) long term administration	due to water imbalance, water accumulation in stomach, *qi xu* "eye dizziness"

		palpitations, distention hypertensive "hat band" headache cold feet
* p. 278	Vitality Combination (*Chen-wu-tang*)	if weak; sp yang *xu* poor GI function
* p. 516	Hoelen 5 Herb Formula (*Wu-ling-san*)	w̄ chronic headache, esp. if thirst also in nephritis
* p. 500	Stephania & Ginseng Combination (*Mu-fang-chi-tang*)	if angina, edema
p. 480	Hoelen, Apricot, & Licorice Comb. (*Fu-ling-hsing-jen-kan-tsao-tang*) hoelen 6 gm apricot seed 4 gm licorice 1 gm	if severe angina
* p. 190	Coptis & Rhubarb Combination	if hypertensive hat band headache, flushed constipation also menopausal
* p. 51	Pueraria Combination (*Ko-ken-tang*)	*tai* yang stage w̄ shoulder stiffness
* p. 76	*Ma-huang-tang*	w̄ no shoulder stiffness or general body ache
* p. 128	Major Bupleurum Comb. (*Ta-chai-hu-tang*)	*shao* yang stage (after 5-7 days of illness) severe chest distress constipation
* p. 340	Bupleurum & Dragon Bone Comb.	if weak pt: insomnia palpitations
* p. 245	Rehmannia 6 Formula (*Liu-wei-ti-huang-wan*)	w̄ chronic kidney infection/nephritis ki yang *xu*
* p. 250	Rehmannia 8 Formula	milder ki yin *xu*
* p. 585	Tang-kuei & Peony Formula	anemia/yin *xu;* dysmenorrhea
* p. 87	Bupleurum & Peony Formula (*Chia-wei-hsiao-yao-san*)	blood congestion dizziness shoulder stiffness tinnitus palpitations dark complexion cold limbs dysmenorrhea

* p. 395	Pinellia & Magnolia Comb. (*Pan-hsia-hou-pu-tang*)	neurotic complaints "stuck in throat feeling" fatigue
* p. 351	Cinnamon & Dragon Bone Comb. (*Kuei-chih-chia-lung-ku-mu-li-tang*)	very weak: ki *xu* neurasthenia/impotence cold in sex organs nocturnal emission spastic rectus abdominis
* p. 105	Pinellia Combination (*Pan-hsia-hsieh-hsin-tang*)	dizziness $\overline{w}$ vomiting/nausea/dry heaves water accumulation in stomach
* p. 190	Coptis & Rhubarb Combination (*San-huang-hsieh-hsin-tang*)	$\overline{w}$ congestion in head constipation
p. 493	Atractylodes & Hoelen Comb. (*Ling-kuei-chu-kan-tang*)	dizziness due to orthostatic hypotension getting up too quickly
p. 511	Alisma Comb. (*Tse-hsieh-tang*)	spinning room vertigo "head dizziness"
* p. 561	Pinellia & Gastrodia Comb. (*Pan-hsia-pai-chu-tien-ma-tang*)	if dizziness accompanied by nausea; and headache
* p. 87	Bupleurum & Peony Formula (*Chia-wei-hsiao-yao-san*)	liver yang rising/contravection menopausal; headache, tinnitus
* p. 343	Bupleurum Formula (*I-kan-san*)	more severe psychological hypersensitivity easily angered insomnia
* p. 250	Rehmannia 8 Formula (*Pa-wei-ti-huang-wan*)	insufficiency of ki *qi*- water (yin *xu*) tinnitus insomnia night sweats
* p. 262	Ginseng & Tang-kuei 10 Formula (*Shih-chuan-ta-pu-tang*) or	anemic irritability insomnia weak limbs prefers not to speak
* p. 425	Ginseng & Longan Comb. (*Kuei-pi-tang*)	severe insomnia hemorrhage, palpitations
* p. 278	Vitality Combination (*Chen-wu-tang*)	insufficient fire in lower heater eye "floaters"

		palpitation P=weak, small
* p. 313	Aconite & G.L. Combination (*Szu-ni-tang*)	more severe weakness red face; pale body diarrhea cold extremities

DYSMENORRHEA

	***XUE-YU*/Oketsu**	**Weak Patient with Blood Stagnancy**
* p. 585	Tang-kuei & Peony Formula (*Tang-kuei-shao-yao-san*)	weak pt, low back pain
* p. 576	Tang-kuei & Gelatin Comb. (*Chiung-kuei-chiao-ai-tang*)	weak & anemic w̄ bleeding
* p. 588	Tang-kuei & Evodia Combination (*Wen-ching-tang*)	weak & cold pt in lower heater heat/dry upper heater
* p. 319	Tang-kuei, Evodia, & Ginger Combination	extreme stagnancy & weak purplish lips/extremities
* p. 423	Cinnamon & Hoelen Formula (*Kuei-chih-fu-ling-wan*)	teenage menstrual complaint with average strength
		Strong Patient with Blood Stasis
* p. 435	Persica & Rhubarb Combination (*Tao-ho-cheng-chi-tang*)	internal heat excess: constipation polyuria
* p. 626	Rhubarb & Moutan Combination (*Ta-huang-mu-tan-pi-tang*)	lower **right** quadrant stagnancy chronic appendicitis watch for rhubarb effect: undigested food in stool
		Chronic, Long Standing Stagnancy
p. 437	Rhubarb & Leech Combination (*Ti-tang-tang*)	strong patient may be too hard on stomach weaker patient
*****p. 423	Cinnamon & Hoelen Formula plus	ANY GYNECOLOGICAL CONDITION
* p. 585	Tang-kuei & Peony Formula	unresponsive or unknown etiology

* p. 87	Bupleurum & Peony Formula (*Chia-wei-hsiao-yao-san*)	emotional swings/irritability only before menses esp. w̄ flushing
	or, if severe	
* p. 343	Bupleurum Formula (*I-kan-san*)	

DYSPNEA

Asthmatic Dyspnea

* p. 43	Minor Blue Dragon Comb. (*Hsiao-ching-lung-tang*)	Strong pt; floating, rapid pulse thin sputum in excess edema
* p. 405	*Shih-ti-tang* (Kaki Combination)	hiccoughs
* p. 405	*Su-tzu-chiang-chi-tang* (Perilla Fruit Comb.)	weak pt; heat upper *jiao* cold lower *jiao*/legs; *shi* pulse good in elderly, dysuria combined lu/ki *xu*
	also/or	
* p. 395	*Pan-hsia-hou-pu-tang* (Pinellia & Magnolia Comb.)	emotional stress/fatigue weak pulse
	with	
p. 300	Licorice & Ginger Comb. (*Kan-tsao-kan-chiang-tang*)	tonifies metabolism/circulation
* p. 128	Major Bupleurum Combination (*Ta-chai-hu-tang*)	chronic asthma in STRONG pt
	with	
* p. 395	Pinellia & Magnolia Comb.	
* p. 401	Mahuang & Magnolia Comb. (*Shen-mi-tang*)	chronic asthma in WEAK pt scanty sputum but persistent cough melancholy soft abdomen
*	Minor Bupleurum Comb.	childhood asthma
	with	
*	Pinellia & Magnolia Comb.	
	Gypsum, Citrus, & Pinellia Comb. (*Wu-hu-erh-chen-tang*)	for prolonged administration
p. 376	Atractylodes & Cardamon Comb. (*Chuan-szu-chun-tzu-tang*)	weak yin *xu* asthma; elderly

"CARDIAC ASTHMA"
Congestive Heart Failure

Page	Formula	Indications
* p. 500	*Mu-fang-chi-tang* (Stephania & Ginseng Combination)	abdominal distention/hardening below heart; edema, flushing up
p. 480	*Fu-ling-hsing-jen-kan-tsao-tang* (Hoelen, Apricot, and Licorice Combination)	severe chest pains to back; submerged, small pulse; severe arteriosclerotic
* p. 556	Hoelen & Schizandra Combination	left side cardiac weakness; lower extremity edema, cyanosis; chill extremities
p. 388	Trichosanthes, Bakeri, (green onion) & Vinegar Combination (*Kua-lou-hsieh-pai-pai-chiu-tang*)	angina w̄ dyspnea, cough
p. 553	*Kua-lou-chih-shih-tang* (Trichosanthes & Chih-shih Combination)	angina w̄ dyspnea- thick sputum, dry mouth; internal heat; **smokers cough
p. 584	Tang-kuei Formula	arteriosclerotic angina w̄ dyspnea
* p. 325	Evodia Combination (*Wu-chu-yu-tang*)	if very weak patient, yang *xu*
p. 161	Gardenia & Soja Combination (*Chih-tzu-shih-tang*)	extremely weak w̄ dyspnea, angina; irritability
p. 389	Trichosanthes, Bakeri, & Pinellia Combination (*Kua-lou-hsieh-pai-pan-hsia-tang*)	severe angina to back; dyspnea; vomiting; weak, irregular (knotted) pulse

EAR INFECTIONS

Chronic Purulent

Page	Formula	Indications
p. 496	Hoelen, Licorice, & Schizandra Comb. (*Ling-kuei wei-kan-tang*)	exudative otitis media; oliguria; upper heat but cold limbs; cardiac hyperfunction; maybe cough, emphysema

hoelen	6 gm
licorice	2 gm
cinnamon	4 gm
schizandra	3 gm

EDEMA

	Formulation	Differentiation
* p. 43	Minor Blue Dragon Combination (*Hsiao-ching-lung-tang*)	"yang edema" upper body/head edema; dry heat localized "bone" pain eyes swollen, puffy Tx: induce sweating diuretics
* p. 81	Major Blue Dragon Combination (*Ta-ching-lung-tang*) if more severe w̄ extreme thirst	
p. 519	Hoelen & Areca Combination (*Wu-pi-yin*)	generalized edema
* p. 293	Astragalus Combination (*Huang-chi-chien-chung-tang*)	"yin edema" ("yin *xue*") lower body edema; diarrhea/oliguria clear to whitish urine pale P – slow generalized diffuse dull pain
* p. 255	Ginseng & Astragalus Comb. (*Pu-chung-i-chi-tang*)	if spleen *xu* predominates diarrhea after eating
* p. 278	Vitality Combination (*Chen-wu-tang*)	exhaustion
* p. 250	Rehmannia 8 Formula (*Pa-wei-ti-huang-wan*)	if kidney *xu* predominates cold extremities; weak
* p. 516	Hoelen 5 Herb Formula (*Wu-ling-san*)	acute glomerulonephritis
* p. 500	Stephania & Ginseng Comb. (*Mu-fang-chi-tang*)	cardiac edema weak; dyspnea edema lower extremities abdomen stiff; subcostal pain indurated orange peel skin
* p. 519	Capillaris Combination (*Yin-chen-hao-tang*)	hepatic edema acute stage jaundice, icterus
* p. 525	Capillaris & Hoelen Formula (*Yin-chen-wu-ling-san*)	liver & kidney disease edema; thirst w̄ vomiting
* p. 585	Tang-kuei & Peony Formula (*Tang-kuei-shao-yao-san*) 1 gm/day	pregnancy edema prevents anemia miscarriage low back pain postpartum edema

	Formula	Indication
* p. 250	Rehmannia 8 Formula (*Pa-wei-ti-huang-wan*)	geriatric (male) edema ki yang *xu*
p. 480	Hoelen, Apricot, & Licorice Comb. (*Fu-ling-hsing-jen-kan-tsao-tang*)	pulmonary edema $\overline{w}$ angina
* p. 205	Hoelen & Alisma Combination (*Fen-hsiao-tang*)	ascites not if abdomen flacid/weak not in weak patient
p. 470	Areca Seed Combination (*Chiu-ping-wu-fu-tang*)	beri-beri edema; alcoholic hypertension; facial edema, heat constipation but cold limbs geriatric malnutrition
* p. 250	Rehmannia 8 Formula (*Pa-wei-ti-huang-wan*)	in weak patient elderly ki yang *xu*
* p. 556	Hoelen & Schizandra Comb. (*Ling-kan-chiang-wei-hsin-jen-tang*)	chronic respiratory disorder
* p. 477	Stephania & Astragalus Comb. (*Fang-chi-huang-chi-tang*)	obese and weak "water obesity" flacid, weak muscles sweating spontaneous pain in knees
* p. 255	Ginseng & Astragalus Comb. (*Pu-chung-i-chi-tang*)	spleen yang *xu* very weak edema dry skin

EXHAUSTION/FATIGUE

	Formula	Indication
* p. 264	Major Four Herb Comb. (*Szu-chun-tzu-tang*)	***Qi* Weakness** (esp. St/Sp *qi xu*) palpitations **poor appetite **dyspnea spont. sweating yellow (sallow) complexion chills P- weak, thin, sinking T- whitish coat
* pl 260	Ginseng & Atractylodes Formula (*Sheng-ling-pai-chu-san*)	chronic gastroenteritis watery diarrhea
* p. 239	Ginseng Nutritive Combination (*Jen-sheng-yang-yung-tang*) or	**Blood (*Xue*) Weakness** dizziness spots in front of eyes blurred vision
* p. 432	Tang-kuei Four Combination	

Formula	Differentiation
(*Szu-wu-tang*) or * p. 425 Ginseng & Longan Combination (*Kuei-pi-tang*) loss appetite no tongue coat	palpitations pale complexion no dyspnea amenorrhea or long intervals between P- thin, weak T- pale
p. 236 Astragalus & Tortoise Shell Formula (TB yin heat) or * p. 199 Phellodendron Combination (*Tzu-yin-chiang-huo-tang*)	**Yin Weakness** fever sensation-maybe cold limbs sticky sweat hemotysis flushed face; irritable; anger nocturnal emissions insomnia poor memory P- fast, thready T- red
* p. 250 Rehmannia Eight Formula (*Pa-wei-ti-huang-wan*) (esp. lower heater-weak, cold limbs) or * p. 264 Major Four Herb Combination (*Szu-chun-tzu-tang*) dry mouth; digestion or	**Yang Weakness** no desire to speak dizzy pale face no appetite chills P- weak, thin, slow T- white coat
* p. 242 Major Six Herb Combination (*Liu-chun-tzu-tang*)	cold limbs, sputum, digestion
p. 437 Rhubarb & Leech Combination (*Ti-tang-tang*) or p. 580 Persica & Eupolyphaga Comb. (*Hsia-yu-hsieh-tang*)	**Stagnant Blood Weakness (*Yu*)** emaciated body but fullness lower abdomen dry skin black around eyes amenorrhea or dysmenorrhea P- irregular, thready "choppy", "tense, wiry" T- purple, black, or red (dark)
p. 253 Lily Combination (*Pai-ho-ku-chin-tang*) lu/ki yin *xu*	**Chronic Infection Exhaustion** (TB) labored cough w̄ exhaustion following dry cough, maybe hemoptysis chest emaciated w̄ pain P- thin T- pale

	Formula	Indication
p. 232	Chin-chiu & Tortoise Shell Formula (*Chin-chiu-pieh-chia-san*) or	high fever; sticky sweat mucoid cough, asthmatic breathing, hemoptysis, insomnia, emaciation P- thin, rapid T-red
p. 273	Aster Combination (*Tzu-wan-tang*)	
p. 273	Aster Combination or	late stage TB: skin pale, woody sleeps, weak cough, asthmatic breathing, feeble voice, red cheeks, lips/face ashen
* p. 537	Ophiopogon Combination (*Mai-men-tung-tang*)	
p. 218	Astragalus & Atractylodes Comb. (*Ching-shu-i-chi-tang*)	summer weight loss/poor appetite with fatigue
* p. 255	Ginseng & Astragalus Comb. (*Pu-chung-i-chi-tang*)	general weak pt; exhaustion due to overwork
* p. 264	Major Four Herb Comb. (*Szu-chun-tzu-tang*)	weakness after eating "exhaustion of the stomach"
* p. 242	Major Six Herb Combination (*Liu-chun-tzu-tang*)	
* p. 262	Ginseng & Tang-kuei 10 Comb. (*Shih-chuan-ta-pu-tang*) or	if with cold limbs poor appetite, digestion
* p. 291	Minor Cinnamon & Peony Comb. (*Hsiao-chien-chung-tang*)	
* p. 260	Ginseng & Atractylodes Formula (*Sheng-ling-pai-chu-san*)	diarrhea/fatigue after eating
* p. 561	Pinellia & Gastrodia Comb. (*Pan-hsia-pai-chu-tien-ma-tang*)	headache/fatigue after eating
p. 218	Astragalus & Atractylodes Comb. (*Ching-shu-i-chi-tang*)	summer diarrhea/fatigue
* p. 278	Vitality Combination (*Chen-wu-tang*)	winter diarrhea/fatigue
* p. 250	Rehmannia Eight Formula (*Pa-wei-ti-huang-wan*)	weak, cold legs predominate with fatigue
	Ji-ming-san	paralysis/edema predominates with fatigue

Ji-ming-san		
areca	4	gm
perilla leaf	1	gm
Citrus reticulata	2.5	gm
platycodon	2.5	gm
fresh ginger	3	gm
chaenomeles	3	gm
evodia	1	gm

* p. 262	Ginseng & Tang-kuei Ten Comb. (*Shih-chuan-ta-pu-tang*)	post-illness weakness; poor recovery
* p. 291	Minor Cinnamon & Peony Comb. (*Hsiao-chien-chung-tang*)	winter: fear cold; summer: weak legs (esp. children of weak constitution)

EXTERNAL INJURY

* p. 415	Musk & Catechu Formula (*Chi-li-san*)	trauma, contusions (*yu*), general pain; not in pregnancy; very expensive
p. 417	Gelatin & Artemisia Four Comb. (*Chiao-ai-szu-wu-tang*)	bleeding caused by external injury; internal bleeding w̄ resulting anemia; purpura
p. 419	Tang-kuei & Persica Comb. (*Fu-yuan-huo-hsieh-tang*)	pain from external injury, contusions
p. 108	Peony & Licorice Combination (*Shao-yao-kan-tsao-tang*) peony 6 gm licorice 6 gm add aconite if severe pain 1 gm	relieves spasm, checks pain
* p. 87	Bupleurum & Peony Formula (*Chia-wei-hsiao-yao-san*)	post surgical syndrome esp. post hysterectomy
* p. 624	Bupleurum & Schizonepeta Comb. (*Shih-wei-pai-tu-tang*)	swelling & inflammation, heat suppuration, lymphadenapathy hypersensitivity
* p. 523	Atractylodes Combination (*Yueh-pi-chia-chu-tang*)	edema from trauma fluid in knee

EYE DISORDERS

p. 598	Lycium, Chrysanthemum, & Rehmannia (6) Formula (*Chi-chu-ti-huang-wan*) or	liver/kidney exhausted w̄ *jing*/blood insuficiency eyes painful dizzy/blurred vision

	Formula	Indication
	30 lycium seeds/day plus Tang-kuei Four Combination	if also severe blood deficiency
* p. 425	Ginseng & Longan Combination (*Kuei-pi-tang*)	heart/spleen weakness w̄ blood deficiency blurred vision palpitations insomnia
* p. 255	Ginseng & Astragalus Comb. (*Pu-chung-i-chi-tang*) eyes painful tired poor appetite	eyes swollen photophobia difficulty blinking- gritty feeling-sticky excessive reading
	Hoelen & Polygala Formula (*Ding-zhi-wan*) 'Calming the Will Pill' ginseng 3 gm polygala 3 gm acorus 3 gm hoelen center (*fu-shen*) 3 gm	myopia with yang *qi* weak
p. 245, 250 p. 85	Rehmannia 6 or 8 Bupleurum, Cinnamon, & Dry Ginger Combination	presbyopia (farsightedness)
		"False Myopia"
* p. 493	Atractylodes & Hoelen Comb. (*Ling-kuei-chu-kan-tang*)	40% - weakness dizziness heavy head (dampness) palpitations gastric water stagnancy possibly vertigo
* p. 516	Hoelen Five Herb Formula (*Wu-ling-san*)	40% - weakness severe thirst sweating diminished urination abdominal palpitations
* p. 291	Minor Cinnamon & Peony Comb. (*Hsiao-chien-chung-tang*)	20%-*tai*-yin weak spastic rectus abdominis nosebleeds
* p. 128 * p. 91 * p. 493	Major Bupleurum Comb. Minor Bupleurum Comb. combined w̄ Hoelen 5 Herb Atractylodes & Hoelen Comb.	

Page	Formula	Indication
* p. 395	Pinellia & Magnolia Comb. or	weakness in stomach meridian
* p. 128	Major/Minor Bupleurum Comb.	
* p. 291	Minor Cinnamon & Peony Comb.	
* p. 250	Rehmannia Eight Comb.	hypertensive myopia
* p. 190	Coptis & Rhubarb (or Scute)	
* p. 128	Major Bupleurum Comb.	
* p. 585	Tang-kuei & Peony Comb.	
* p. 340	Bupleurum & Dragon Bone Comb.	
* p. 87	Bupleurum & Peony Comb.	female myopia
* p. 423	Cinnamon & Hoelen Comb.	
* p. 435	Persica & Rhubarb Comb.	
* p. 319	Tang-kuei, Evodia, & Ginger Comb.	

KERATITIS (Corneal inflammation)

Page	Formula	Indication
* p. 599	Gardenia & Vitex Comb. (*Hsi-kan-ming-mu-tang*) 'Cleanse the Liver & Brighten Eye Tea'	w̄ conjunctivitis strong pt
* p. 271	Scute Combination (*Tzu-sheng-tung-erh-tang*)	weak pt
* p. 250	Rehmannia Eight Formula	cataracts
* p. 183	Ginseng & Gypsum Combination (*Jen-sheng-pai-hu-tang*)	photophobia w̄ itching
* p. 262	Ginseng & Tang-kuei 10 Comb. (*Shih-chuan-ta-pu-tang*) "Wind Evil attacking a weak patient"	heavy eyelids weak/dizziness numbness of eyelid (*myasthenia gravis*)

Excess Tearing

'COLD TEARS'

Page	Formula	Indication
* p. 262	Ginseng & Tang-kuei 10 Comb. (*Shih-chuan-ta-pu-tang*) or Rehmannia and Achyranthes Formula (*Yu-kuei-wan*) ™ 'Pill of Left (Ki) Tonification' (Yang) rehmannia, prepared 8 gm dioscorea 4 gm achyranthes 3 gm	'cold' tears: ki *xu* *jing/xue* exhaustion, often w̄ emphysema bronchitis/TB thin, watery tears no pain; no redness wind aggravates Tx: tonify *qi/xue* to nourish kidney yin tonify *qi/jing* to

	lycium 4 gm deer horn gelatin 4 gm tortoise shell gelatin 4 gm cuscuta 4 gm	replenish kidney yang
* p. 78	Morus & Chrysanthemum Combination (*Sang-chu-yin*)	'hot' tears: liver heat wind evil (onion effect) inflammatory w̄ redness swelling, pain thick concentrated tears photophobia heat flush on tearing
	Bamboo Leaf and Bupleurum Comb. (*Chu-yeh-hsieh-ching-tang*) 'Bamboo leaf Purging/Cleansing Tea' bupleurum, coptis gardenia, rhubarb *chiang-huo*, hoelen cimicifuga, peony licorice, alisma scute, cassia plantago, bamboo leaf equal parts	pustular, swollen eye infection 'stye' or chelazion
* p. 190	Coptis & Rhubarb Combination (*San-huang-hsieh-hsin-tang*)	if hard internal core of swelling
* p. 631	Gleditsia Combination (*Tuo-li-hsiao-tu-yin*)	w̄ suppuration strong pt
* p. 239	Ginseng Nutritive Combination (*Jen-sheng-yang-yung-tang*) or	weak pt
p. 631	Astragalus & Platycodon Formula	

Dry Eyes

p. 598	Lycium, Chrysanthemum, & Rehmannia (6) (*Chi-chu-ti-huang-wan*)	itching, painful, gritty blood/yin weak overwork lack of sleep

Photophobia

* p. 609	Schizonepeta & Siler Formula (*Ching-fang-pai-tu-san*) 'Purge Wind, Remove Toxin Powder' Vit B_2 deficiency adrenal weakness	itching, painful profuse tears blurred vision redness

Chronic Dacryocystitis

* p. 523	Atractylodes Combination (*Yueh-pi-chia-chu-tang*) excessive tearing	Lacrimal sac inflammation due to accumulated heat he/sp yin *xu* attacking eye exogenous wind-heat (bacterial/viral) excessive thinking/anxiety
* p. 402	Tang-kuei 16 Formula (*Shih-liu-wei-liu-chi-yin*)	if pustular and/or conjunctivitis

FEVER

Wind-Chill

* p. 76	Mahuang Combination (*Ma-huang-tang*)	*tai* yang: chills and fever, runny nose, general ache no sweating strong pt, great irritability
* p. 63	Cinnamon Combination (*Kuei-chih-tang*)	weak pt: spontaneous sweating
* p. 72	Mahuang & Asarum Comb. (*Ma-huang-fu-tzu-hsi-hsin-tang*)	weak pt: no sweating; extremities cold
* p. 41	Cyperus & Perilla Formula (*Hsiang-su-san*) (food poisoning)	GI weakness, distress, weak pt chest congestion, stiff shoulders tinnitus, nausea, heavy head watery vomit, food accumulation T- yellow coat
* p. 609	Schizonepeta & Siler Formula (*Ching-fang-pai-tu-san*)	fever but chill precedes and predominates, esp. if suppuration septicemia from skin infections

Wind-Heat

* p. 51	Pueraria Combination (*Ko-ken-tang*)	*tai* yang: strong pt/no sweating stiff shoulders, respiratory congestion, possible diarrhea
* p. 78	Morus & Chrysanthemum (*Sang-chu-yin*) or	sore throat, dry harsh cough, thirst red eyes, dehydration Tx: cooling/moisturizing
* p. 83	Lonicera & Forsythia Formula (*Yin-chiao-san*)	mild sore throat, irritability

Formula	Indication
	Tidal Fever
* p. 91 Minor Bupleurum Comb. (*Hsiao-chai-hu-tang*)	*shao* yang: alternating chill/fever decreased appetite; chest distress infra-costal margin tender T–thick, yellow, brown, white coat bitter taste in mouth
	Yang *Ming* Fever
p. 185 Gypsum Combination (*Pai-hu-tang*) =White Tiger Tea for severe fever gypsum 15 gm anemarrhena 5 gm licorice 2 gm brown rice 8 gm	½ *biao* (respiratory/skin) ½ *li* (digestive) vomiting; bitter taste chest distress fever w̄ thirst (do not give if no thirst) skin itching/heat big fever big pulse big abdomen big thirst
**p. 183 Ginseng & Gypsum Comb. (*Pai-hu-chia-jen-sheng-tang*) for less severe fever	also must have thirst weaker patient
p. 145 Major Rhubarb Combination (*Ta-cheng-chi-tang*)	high fever w̄ constipation, thirst sweating, delirium, gasping T- dark coat P- deep but firm
p. 220 Bamboo Leaves & Gypsum Combination (*Chu-yeh-shih-kao-tang*)	extremely high fever in weak pt yin *xu* heat also: fever of unknown origin dry skin, night sweats

GASTRIC DISTRESS

Formula	Indication
***Shao* Yang Middle Heater Heat**	**Gastroenteritis**
p. 105 Pinellia Combination (*Pan-hsia-hsieh-hsin-tang*)	vomiting gastric ulcers diarrhea or constipation

Page	Formulation	Differentiation
		"water in the stomach" borborygmus/nausea
p. 98	Coptis Combination (*Huang-lien-tang*)	chest/stomach nausea stomach chill/clear vomitus bad breath, hyperacidity abdomen cold to touch cold clammy sweat acute food poisoning
p. 103	Pinellia & Licorice Comb. (*Kan-tsao-hsieh-hsin-tang*)	GI distress w̄ emotional distress "*qi* disruption"-hypersensitive dry heaves, diarrhea
p. 110	Pinellia & Ginger Comb. (*Sheng-chiang-hsieh-hsin-tang*) add: *Prunus mume* zanthoxylum	stagnant food/bad breath nausea, diarrhea if excessive saliva
p. 395	Pinellia & Magnolia Comb. (*Pan-hsia-hou-pu-tang*)	esophageal constriction "stuck in throat" hysterical neurotic component esp. w̄ insomnia
p. 555	Pinellia & Gardenia Comb. (*Li-ke-tang*)	difficulty swallowing esophageal cancer
p. 212	Magnolia & Ginger Comb. (*Ping-wei-san*)	nausea, gastric fullness after eating/hyperacidity
p. 366	Cardamon & Fennel Comb. (*An-chung-san*)	more severe pain/gastroenteritis w̄ nervous constitution soda substitute
p. 325	Evodia Combination (*Wu-chu-yu-tang*)	severe headaches w̄ vomiting esp. women weak w̄ chill
p. 255	Ginseng & Astragalus Comb. (*Pu-chung-i-chi-tang*)	gastroptosis-prolapse weak pt
p. 242	Major 6 Herb Combination (*Liu-chun-tzu-tang*)	poor appetite, cold extremities
p. 254	Pinellia & Ginseng Comb. (*Pan-hsieh-liu-chun-tzu-tang*)	gastric and/or duodenal ulcers

Diarrhea

Page	Formulation	Differentiation
p. 105	Pinellia Combination (*Pan-hsia-hsieh-hsin-tang*)	acute diarrhea

p. 278	Vitality Combination (*Chen-wu-tang*)	Chronic diarrhea
p. 516	Hoelen 5 Herb Formula (*Wu-ling-san*)	children's diarrhea
p. 122	Pueraria, Coptis, & Scute Comb. (*Ko-ken-huang-lien-huang-chin-tang*)	amebic, bacillary dysentery w̄/pus, blood in stools

Habitual Constipation

p. 128	Major Bupleurum Comb. (*Ta-chai-hu-tang*)	habitual constipation strong pt- more chest distress abdominal distention shoulder stiffness hypertension
p. 190	Coptis & Rhubarb Comb. (*San-huang-hsieh-hsin-tang*)	habitual constipation strong pt- more internal heat flushing, nervous, anger emotional instability chest distress
p. 535	Apricot Seed & Linum Formula (*Ma-tzu-jen-wan*)	habitual constipation weak pt, chronic; elderly dry skin
p. 141	Minor Cinnamon & Peony Comb. (*Hsiao-chien-chung-tang*)	habitual constipation children
p. 585	Tang-kuei & Peony Comb. (*Tang-kuei-shao-yao-san*)	habitual constipation pregnancy menopause

Vomiting/Nausea

(p. 57)	Pinellia & Hoelen Formula (*Hsiao-pan-hsia-chia-fu-ling-tang*)	pregnancy nausea/morning sickness
p. 516	Hoelen 5 Herb Formula (*Wu-ling-san*)	stomach flu, esp. vomiting after drinking water
p. 626	Rhubarb & Moutan Comb.	appendicitis

Dichotomous Key of Symptoms

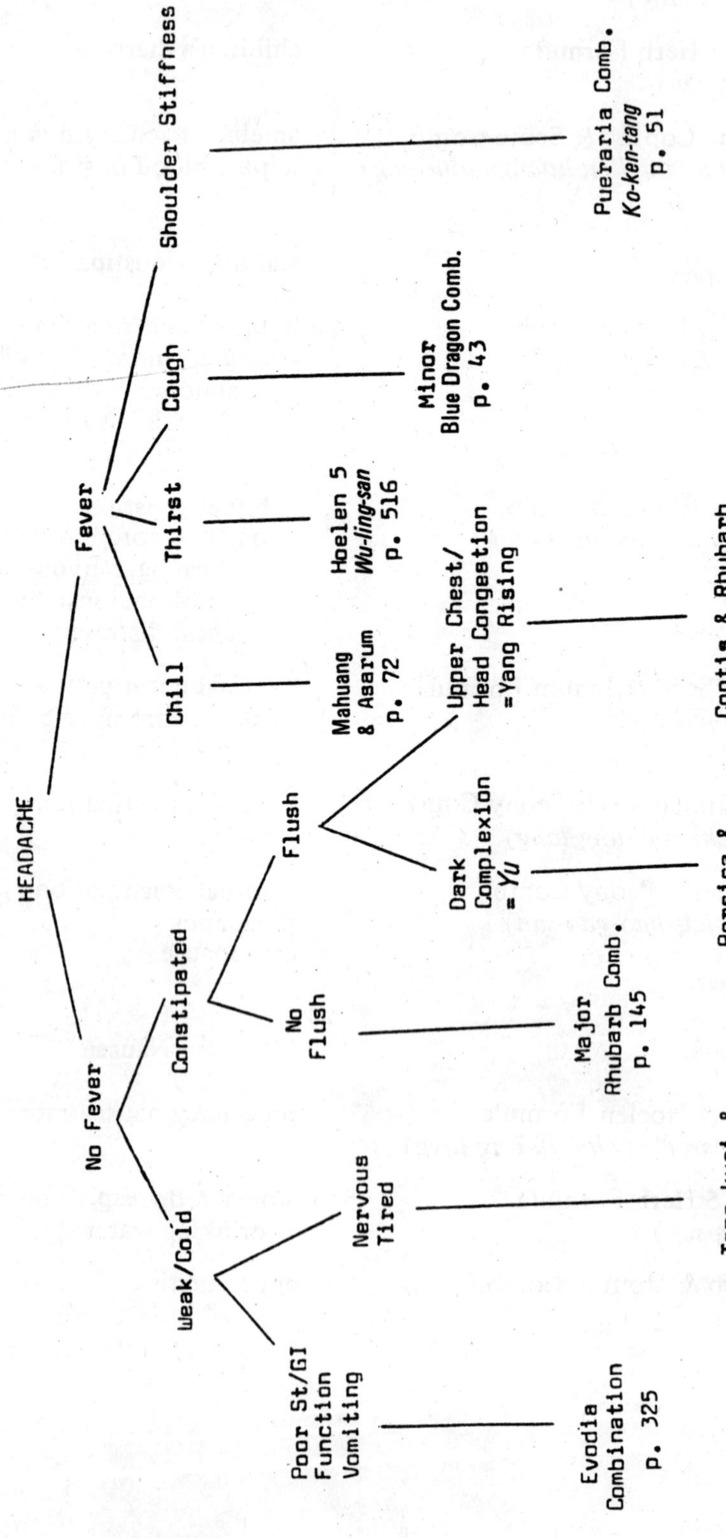

HEADACHES

	Formula	Indication
* p. 325	*Wu-chu-yu-tang* (Evodia Combination)	coldness in stomach w̄ vomiting yang *xu*
* p. 585	*Tang-kuei-shao-yao-san* (Tang-kuei & Peony Formula)	weak patients w̄ dysmenorrhea, anemia
p. 145	*Ta-cheng-chi-tang* (Major Rhubarb Combination)	constipation, high fever, delirium
p. 435	*Tao-ho-cheng-chi-tang* (Persica & Rhubarb Combination)	dysmenorrhea, constipation, left lower quadrant pain
* p. 190	*San-huang-hsieh-hsin-tang* (Coptis & Rhubarb Combination)	constipation, flushed face, irritability
* p. 72	*Ma-huang-fu-tzu-hsi-hsin-tang* (Mahaung & Asarum Combination)	fever/chills, cold extremities
* p. 516	*Wu-ling-san* (Hoelen Five Herb Formula)	fever with thirst, dysuria
* p. 43	*Hsiao-ching-lung-tang* (Minor Blue Dragon Combination)	wind-chill cough; clear nasal secretion
* p. 51	*Ko-ken-tang* (Pueraria Combination)	with shoulder/neck stiffness
* p. 561	*Pan-hsia-pai-chu-tien-ma-tang* (Pinellia & Gastrodia Combination)	chronic headache w̄ dizziness cold extremities/vomiting
p. 493	*Ling-kuei-chu-kan-tang* (Atractylodes & Hoelen Comb.)	w̄ dizziness/vertigo/palpitations nervousness; poor GI function
* p. 386	*Kou-teng-san* (Gambir Formula)	hypertensive headache ringing in ears
* p. 343	*I-kan-san* (Bupleurum Formula)	severe menopausal/anger neurotic hypersensitivity
* p. 87	*Chia-wei-hsiao-yao-san* (Bupleurum & Peony Formula)	mild menopausal complaints irritability, weakness
* p. 40	*Chuan-chiung-cha-tiao-san* (Cnidium & Tea Formula)	migraine (wind-heat)
* p. 255	*Pu-chung-i-chi-tang* (Ginseng & Astragalus Comb.)	*qi xu* weakness: emptiness in head chilled, palpitations, anorexia
* p. 433	*Szu-wu-tang* (Tang-kuei Four Combination)	anemic headache (mild) pale; dizzy; palpitation worse in PM dry skin

	Formula	Differentiation
* p. 248	*Pa-chen-tang* (Tang-kuei & Ginseng 8 Comb.)	both *xue* & *qi xu* general weakness; anorexia
* p. 212	*Ping-wei-san* (Magnolia & Ginger Comb.)	stomach heat (food accumulation) headache; constipation; foul breath
p. 212	*Pao-ho-wan* (Citrus & Crataegus Formula)	severe stomach heat headache
* p. 343	*I-kan-san* (Bupleurum Formula)	vascular migraine headache to vertex liver yang rising; red eyes
* p. 561	*Pan-hsia-pai-chu-tien-ma-tang* (Pinellia & Gastrodia Comb.)	severe damp/phlegm accumulation headache- heaviness/dizziness
* p. 521	*Yin-chen-wu-ling-san* (Capillaris & Hoelen Formula)	mild damp/phlegm headache combined ki/liver disease w̄/jaundice
p. 598	*Chi-chu-ti-huang-wan* (Lycium, Chrysanthemum, and Rehmannia Formula)	ki *qi xu* headache emptiness/tinnitus/blurred vision
* p. 561	Pinellia & Gastrodia Comb. (*Pan-hsia-pai-chu-tien-ma-tang*) dispel hidden water chronic: 2-6 month Tx	headache w̄ dizziness (chronic) cold extremities vomiting, weak poor GI function (*li hsui*) P- weak but rapid
* p. 325	Evodia Combination (*Wu-chu-yu-tang*)	w̄ more severe vomiting migraines
p. 493	Atractylodes & Hoelen Comb. (*Ling-kuei-chu-kan-tang*)	w̄ nervousness/palpitations hyperventilation/vertigo flushing up in elderly

HYPERTENSIVE HEADACHES
(worse on waking)

	Formula	Differentiation
* p. 386	Gambir Formula (*Kou-teng-san*)	increase peripheral vasodilation sedative (cooling) weak pt w̄ poor liver function insomnia/irritable
* p. 190	Coptis & Rhubarb Comb. (*San-huang-hsieh-hsin-tang*)	severe congestion in head with tinnitus (atherosclerotic) flushing/anger esp. if on Western medication

VASCULAR HEADACHES
(often provoked by anger)

Formula	Indication
* p. 343 Minor Bupleurum Formula (*I-kan-san*) 2x, 3x dosage ok	neurotic hypersensitivity irritable bruxism insomnia fear, panic, terror/weak pt menopausal fear of social contact
* p. 87 Bupleurum & Peony Formula (*Chia-wei-hsiao-yao-san*) plus 4 gm cyperus	if not as severe; slight irritability for women easily upset w̄ headaches
* p. 40 Cnidium & Tea Formula (*Chuan-chiung-cha-tiao-san*)	migraine and unknown etiology wind-heat

HEARING LOSS

Formula	Indication
* p. 51 *Ko-ken-tang* (Pueraria Combination) add if purulent discharge from ear: platycodon 2 gm gypsum 10 gm	acute hearing loss due to pathological heat
* p. 41 Cyperus & Perilla Formula (*Hsiang-su-san*)	*tai yang* cold

CHRONIC

Formula	Indication
* p. 190 Coptis & Rhubarb Combination (*San-huang-hsieh-hsin-tang*)	constipation; arteriosclerosis atherosclerosis high fat diet internal heat, strong pt
* p. 175 Coptis & Scute Combination (*Huang-lien-chieh-tu-tang*)	as above but no constipation
* p. 91 Minor Bupleurum Combination (*Hsiao-chai-hu-tang*)	chronic ear infection w̄ purulent exudate (otorrhea)
* p. 631 Gleditsia Combination (*Tuo-li-hsiao-tu-yin*)	if weaker patient; more chronic otorrhea non-responsive to other Tx

* p. 604	Astragalus & Platycodon Formula (*Chien-chin-nei-tuo-san*)	if severe or prolonged depleted already weak pt
* p. 291	Minor Cinnamon & Peony Combination (*Hsiao-chien-chung-tang*)	children or fatigued pt w̅ GI dysfunction
extra	*Kuei-chi-chien-chung-tang* = Minor Cinnamon and Peony Comb. plus *tang-kuei* 1.5 gm astragalus 1.5 gm	for extremely weak patient
* p. 250	Rehmannia 8 Formula (*Pa-wei-ti-huang-wan*)	hearing loss due to excessive sex; debility (weak legs) tonic for ki yang *xu*
* p. 245	Rehmannia 6 Formula (*Liu-wei-ti-huang-wan*)	tonic for ki yin *xu* flushed, feverish but weak w̅/night sweats

HEMORRHAGE

p. 613	Cimicifuga Combination (*I-tzu-tang*) avoid spicy food alcohol	hemorrhoids dull aching anus intense itching bleeding, constipation
p. 255	Ginseng & Astragalus Comb. (*Pu-chung-i-chi-tang*)	severe hemorrhoids in weak patients
p. 634	Lithospermum Ointment (*Tzu-yun-kao*) and/or Topical Vitamin E 2x a day aloe vera gel on gauze pad calendula serate ointment hypræstis (goldenseal) serate	topical for anal fissure/hemorrhoids
p. 83	Lonicera & Forsythia Comb. (*Yin-chiao-san*)	nosebleeding upper heater wind-heat cough/dry nose headache/thirst T- red w̅ white coat
p. 78	Morus & Chrysanthemum Comb. plus moutan imperata	

Page	Formula	Indication
p. 201	Rehmannia & Gypsum Comb. (*Yu-nu-chien*)	nosebleeding yang *ming* heat in strong pt thirst foul breath constipation T- yellow coat P- big & fast
p. 181	Gentiana Combination (*Lung-tan-hsieh-kan-tang*) plus bupleurum 3 gm peony 3 gm add: scrophularia 3 gm ophiopogon 3 gm	nosebleeding liver fire flaring upward strong headache/dizziness/vertigo dry mouth anger T- red
also:	*Tang-kuei-lung-huei-wan* ™ (Tang-kuei, Gentiana, and Aloe Formula)	nosebleeding due to liver fire
p. 170	Rhinoceros & Rehmannia Comb. (*Hsi-chiao-ti-huang-tang*)	continuous epistaxis blood heat end stage leukemia
p. 201	Rehmannia & Gypsum Comb. (*Yu-nu-chien*) plus mirabilitum 1 gm rhubarb 1 gm if severe constipation	**Gingival Bleeding** due to stomach fire flaring up halitosis constipation gingivitis P- thin but fast
p. 177	Sweet Combination (*Kan-lu-yin*)	gums painful and bleeding **no halitosis**
p. 173	Morus & Lycium Combination (*Hsieh-pai-san*) or *Sang-hsiang-tang* morus leaf 3 gm apricot seed 4.5 gm gardenia 3 gm adenophora 6 gm fritillary 3 gm prepared black soybean 3 gm peach skin 3 gm or *Szu-sheng-wan* fresh lotus leaf 9 gm	**Hemoptysis** wind evil w̄ dry heat throat, mouth, nose dry/itchy headache, fever P- floating & fast

fresh artemisia leaf	9 gm	
fresh thuja leaf	9 gm	
fresh rehmannia	9 gm	
plus indigo	2 gm	liver fire burns the lungs
clam shell	2 gm	lateral costal pain
moutan	2 gm	headache/irritable
scute	2 gm	P- fast, tight

Common Hemorrhage Formula:

Shih-fei-san ("Ten Ash Powder")

cirsium	3 gm
segetum	3 gm
lotus leaf	3 gm
thuja leaf	3 gm
imperata	3 gm
rubia	3 gm
rhubarb	3 gm
gardenia	3 gm
trachycarpus	3 gm
moutan	3 gm

9 mg/dose

p. 175	Coptis & Scute Comb. (*Huang-lien-chieh-tu-tang*)	gastric hemorrhage melena
p. 190	Coptis & Rhubarb Comb. (*San-huang-hsieh-hsin-tang*)	vomiting blood due to stomach heat accumulation violet red clotted blood abdominal pain red lips halitosis heartburn constipation T- yellow coat P- slippery; fast
p. 190	Coptis & Rhubarb Comb. plus gentiana moutan gardenia	vomiting blood due to liver fire rising heart irritable angry bitter taste painful flanks insomnia dreams T- red P- tight, fast, wiry

Coughing Blood

p. 78 Morus & Chrysanthemum Comb.
plus lotus leaf
imperata
bamboo skin

wind-heat attacking lungs
dry throat/headache/fever
violet-red or thin red blood
P–floating, fast

p. 593 Adenophora & Ophiopogon Comb.
plus rehmannia
moutan
pumice (porites)

or

p. 253 Lily Combination

yin-weak/fire & inflammation
high fever
dry cough/dry throat
T–red
P–thin & fast

'Occult' Fecal Blood

p. 425 Ginseng & Longan Combination
(*Kuei-pi-tang*)

Weak & Cold pt
dark-violet blood follows stool
fatigue
speaks little
abdominal pain
T- thin (*xue xu*)
P- tight

p. 420 Fu-lung-kan Combination
(*Huang-tu-tang*)

or

Shih-fei-san
"Ten-Ash Powder"

see previous page

Phaseolus and Tang-kuei Formula
(*Chih-hsiao-tou-tang-kuei-san*)
5.4 liter phaseolus
90 gm *tang-kuei*
2 gm/dose

damp-heat
thin-red or turbid blood prior to stool
T- yellow, greasy
P- slippery, fast

or

Sophora Flower Formula
(*Huai-hua-san*)

sophora flower	7.5 gm
schizonepeta	7.5 gm
thuja	7.5 gm
chih-ko	7.5 gm

or

Hsiung-lien-wan
picrorhiza 60 gm
cooked w̄ 2 feet male pig intestines

Urinary Bleeding

p. 196 Rehmannia & Akebia Formula
(*Tao-chih-san*)
plus gardenia
dianthus
pine resin

or

* p. 502 Dianthus Formula
(*Pa-cheng-san*)

strong pt/small intestine fire
urethritis w̄ burning (needle-like)
weak but irritable
insomnia
dry mouth
swollen tongue
T- yellow coat
P- fast

* p. 87 Bupleurum & Peony Comb.
(*Chia-wei-hsiao-yao-san*)

or

Tang-kuei-lung-hwei-wan ™

or

* p. 181 Gentiana Combination
(*Lung-tan-hsieh-kan-tang*)
plus moutan
Curcuma aromatica (tumeric)

strong pt/liver fire burning inside
needle-like pain flanks
lower abdomen
bitter taste
deafness or difficult hearing
reddish urine
tidal fever
P- tight wiry

Hsiao-chi-yin-tzu

rehmannia	12 gm
akebia	1.5 gm
baked licorice	1.5 gm
cirsium	1.5 gm
lotus root	1.5 gm
typha	1.5 gm
tang-kuei	1.5 gm
talc	1.5 gm
gardenia	1.5 gm

strong pt/heat accumulation
lower heater
drops of turbid blood
following urine w̄ pain

or

* p. 472 Polyporus Combination
(*Chu-ling-tang*)

acute cystitis w̄/hematuria
dysuria

Excessive Sex Injures the Kidney

Ku-lou-er-sheng-kao™

deer antler	20 gm
tortoise shell	10 gm
lycium seed	2 gm
ginseng	1 gm

10 gm/dose

blood in urine without pain
mental exhaustion
dizziness
floaters in eyes
low back discomfort

	Liu-wei-ah-chiao-yin TM = Rehmannia-6 plus gelatin	if yin *xu* heat/weakness anemia, night sweats
	Lu-chiao-chiao-wan TM deer antler 15 gm gelatin myrrh 9 gm human hair ash 9 gm white imperata juice to form pills	if yang *xu*
p. 245	Rehmannia 6 Formula plus *Sheng-mai-san* ginseng 15 gm ophiopogon 9 gm schizandra 6 gm	**Lu/Ki Weakness** dry mouth low back pain
	or	
p. 250	Rehmannia 8 Formula	
	Yu-hsieh-wan astragalus 5-10 gm ginseng 5-10 gm	**Spleen Not Controlling Blood** thrombocytopenic purpura fatigue anorexia T- thin, pale P- weak
		Uterine Hemorrhage
p. 170	Rhinoceros & Rehmannia Comb. (*Hsi-chiao-ti-huang-tang*) *Xi-jiao-di-huang-tang* or *Huai-hua-san* (see occult fecal blood)	**Blood-Heat** sudden onset profuse continuous deep red flow irritable thirst dizziness anxiety insomnia P- huge, fast T- red; yellow dry coat
	Tu-sheng-tang 8 gm/dose Korean red ginseng or	***Qi* Exhaustion** internal hemorrhage thin red blood dizzy or unconscious or blind non-responsive dyspnea yellow face; pale P- thin, weak almost stopped
p. 255	Ginseng & Astragalus Comb. (*Pu-chung-i-chi-tang*)	

p. 239 Ginseng Nutritive Combination
(*Jen-sheng-yang-yung-tang*)
dyspnea
hair loss
dry skin

Injury from Overwork
clear red flow
fatigue w̄ weak extremities
pale
T- thin w̄ yellowish coat
P- big but hollow pulse

p. 262 Ginseng & Tang-kuei 10 Comb.
(*Shih-chuan-ta-pu-tang*)

extremely weak;
poor digestion

p. 432 Tang-kuei 4 Combination

general anemia/menstrual

p. 425 Ginseng & Longan Combination

anemia w̄ cardiac hyperfunction
poor memory

p. 170 Rhinoceros & Rehmannia Comb.
(*Hsi-chiao-ti-huang-tang*)

or

p. 87 Bupleurum & Peony Formula
(*Chia-wei-hsiao-yao-san*)

***Qi* Stagnation/Accumulation (*Yu*)**
blood clots, strong pt
flank & lower abdominal pain
anger/depression
bitter taste
wiry pulse
T- red w̄ yellow coat

Uterine Hemorrhage

p. 583 *Shih-hsiao-san*
= Pteropus & Typha (Bulrush)
3 gm each
added to
Fu-shou-san
(Buddha's Hand Powder)

tang-kuei	9 gm
cnidium	6 gm

6 gm/dose

Stagnant Blood (*Yu*)
violet, clotted blood
lower abdominal pain
that decrease with flow
T- normal w̄ purple spots
P- knotted, choppy

Postpartum Hemorrhage

p. 267 Tang-kuei & Astragalus Comb.
(*Tang-kuei-pu-hsieh-tang*)

tang-kuei	6 gm
astragalus	30 gm

or

Ku-sheng-tang
8 gm dose Korean ginseng

or

anemia
dizziness
eye floaters
pale
dry heaves
cold extremities/cold sweat
maybe unconsciousness
P- thin, hollow

* p. 583	Tang-kuei & Ginger Combination (*Sheng-hua-tang*) *Shih-hsiao-san* plus ophicalcite	***Xue Yu*** **– Blood Stagnation** placental retention lower abdominal pain fullness below heart irritability vomiting purplish face T- purple

General Anti-hemorrhagic Formulas:

1. Coptis & Scute Formulas – upper body heat syndromes w̄ hemorrhage inflammation
2. Rehmannia & Peony Formulas – lower body stagnant blood and/or anemia w̄ hemorrhage
3. Ginseng & Hoelen Formulas – severe anemia from/with hemorrhage

Any Sudden External Hemorrhage

* Single Dose 8 gm (¼ oz.) American ginseng or		cold extremities cold sweat (call emergency paramedics)
* p. 311	Ginger, Licorice, and Aconite w̄ Ginseng (2 gm) Combination (*Szu-ni-chia-jen-sheng-tang*)	if P- weak: easy to cure if P- big & fast: poor prognosis (yin turning to yang before death) if hemorrhage and night sweats: do not use aconite if hemorrhage and sudden exhaustion; combination not use Tang-kuei 4
* p. 255	Ginseng & Astragalus Comb. (*Pu-chung-i-chi-tang*) plus aconite 1 gm	dyspnea, exhaustion, spontaneous sweating
* p. 287	Aconite, Ginseng, & Ginger Comb. (*Fu-tzu-li-chung-tang*)	if diarrhea vomiting exhaustion P- thin/small if extremely weak, do not use rehmannia coptis

Hemoptysis/Hematoemesis

	Formulation	Indication
* p. 537	Ophiopogon Combination (*Mai-men-tung-tang*) plus rehmannia 3 gm gelatin 3 gm coptis 3 gm	dry cough w̄ blood
* p. 85	Bupleurum, Cinnamon, & Ginger Combination (*Chai-hu-kuei-chih-kan-chiang-tang*)	phlegm cough w̄ blood (esp. if TB)
* p. 175	Coptis & Scute Combination (*Huang-lien-chieh-tu-tang*)	vomiting blood
	or	
* p. 190	Coptis & Rhubarb Combination (*San-huang-hsieh-hsin-tang*)	esp. if TB
	Fu-pi-sheng-mai-tang aster 2 gm astragalus 2 gm schizandra 1.5 gm licorice 1.5 gm *tang-kuei* 4 gm bletilla 4 gm ophiopogon 6 gm peony 3 gm	if TB & anorexia/dyspnea
p. 170	Rhinoceros & Rehmannia Combination (*Hsi-chiao-ti-huang-tang*)	if ambiguous abdominal symptoms in weak pt
* p. 435	Persica & Rhubarb Combination (*Tao-ho-cheng-chi-tang*) cold limbs dry mouth and/or constipation	female w̄ vicarious menstruation strong pt w̄ flushing up stagnant blood
* p. 423	Cinnamon & Hoelen Formula (*Kuei-chih-fu-ling-wan*) milder pain	
	Po-yeh-tang plus moxa biota (thuja) 3 gm dry ginger 3 gm *Artemisia vulgaris* 5 gm cooked in 1 liter water	if no other formula works

Epistaxis (nosebleed)

	Formulation	Indication
* p. 76	Mahuang Combination (*Ma-huang-tang*)	w̄ common cold

	Formula	Indication
* p. 291	Minor Cinnamon & Peony Comb. (*Hsiao-chien-chung-tang*)	in weak children

Fecal Blood

	Formula	Indication
* p. 439	Tang-kuei & Gardenia Comb. (*Wen-ching-yin*)	Continuous Bleeding in stool
* p. 295	Ginseng and Ginger Combination (*Li-chung-tang/Jen-sheng-tang*)	over 1 week (rule out cancer)
	or	
* p. 242	Major Six Herb Combination (*Liu-chun-tzu-tang*)	
p. 187	Anemone Combination (*Pai-tou-weng-tang*)	frank red blood in stool w̄ high fever, tenesmus
* p. 175	Coptis & Scute Comb.	if induced by alcohol
	Fu-lung-kan-tang	if blood follows stool

Hematuria

	Formula	Indication
* p. 576	Tang-kuei & Gelatin Comb. (*Chiung-kuei-chiao-ai-tang*)	
* p. 425	Ginseng & Longan Combination (*Kuei-pi-tang*)	if severe anemia
* p. 472	Polyporus Combination (*Chu-ling-tang*)	burning dysuria with anemia
	and	
* p. 433	Tang-kuei Four Combination (*Szu-wu-tang*)	

Excessive and/or Prolonged Menstrual Bleeding (also applies to Hemorrhoidal Bleeding)

	Formula	Indication
* p. 576	Tang-kuei & Gelatin Comb. (*Chiung-kuei-chiao-ai-tang*)	if anemic and cold
* p. 439	Tang-kuei & Gardenia Comb. (*Wen-ching-yin*)	if heat and skin symptoms

	Page	Formula	Indication
	p. 317	Tang-kuei, Cinnamon, & Peony Comb. (*Tang-kuei-chien-chung-tang*) plus rehmannia 2 gm, gelatin 2 gm	if initial menses (menarche)
*	p. 190	Coptis & Rhubarb Comb.	if no results
*	p. 435	Persica & Rhubarb Comb.	if still no results
*	p. 423	Cinnamon & Hoelen Formula (*Kuei-chih-fu-ling-wan*)	uterine fibroid bleeding (symptomatic control–strong pt)
*	p. 576	Tang-kuei & Gelatin Comb. (*Chiung-kuei-chiao-ai-tang*)	if weak pt
	p. 573	Cinnamon & Persica Comb. (*Che-tsung-yin*)	uterine cancer bleeding
*	p. 439	Tang-kuei & Gardenia Comb. (*Wen-ching-yin*)	menopausal bleeding/yin *xu* heat

Postpartum Hemorrhage

	Page	Formula	Indication
*	p. 576	Tang-kuei & Gelatin Comb.	
*	p. 423	Cinnamon & Hoelen Comb.	if due to placental retention, ectopic pregnancy
		and/or	
*	p. 435	Persica & Rhubarb Comb.	

Post Hemorrhage Anemia

	Page	Formula	Indication
*	p. 425	Ginseng & Longan Combination (*Kuei-pi-tang*)	weak w̄ insomnia, palpitations, poor memory
		or	
	p. 427	Tang-kuei & Atractylodes Comb. (*Lien-chu-yin*)	

Cerebral Hemorrhage

	Page	Formula	Indication
*	p. 190	Coptis & Rhubarb Combination	
*	p. 439	Tang-kuei & Gardenia Comb.	ocular/retinal bleeding

HERPES

* p. 181	*Lung-tan-hsieh-kan-tang* (Gentiana Combination)	"dry" genital; red dot/papule raised strong pt
p. 551	*Er-chen-tang* (Citrus & Pinellia Comb.)	"wet" weaker pt
	or	
* p. 516	*Wu-ling-san* (Hoelen 5 Herb Formula)	
* p. 624	*Shih-wei-pai-tu-tang* (Bupleurum & Schizonepeta) plus forsythia & coix	pustular *Herpes zoster*
* p. 51	*Ko-ken-tang* (Pueraria Comb.)	acute stage IF FEVER
* p. 91	*Hsiao-chai-hu-tang* (Minor Bupleurum Comb.)	to 2nd week
* p. 128	*Ta-chai-hu-tang* (Major Bupleurum Comb.)	acute stage if constipation
* p. 278	*Chen-wu-tang* (Vitality Combination)	chronic
* p. 624	*Shih-wei-pai-tu-tang* (Bupleurum & Schizonepeta Comb.)	chronic getting worse add 3 gm forsythia
* p. 183	*Pai-hu-chia-jen-sheng-tang* (Ginseng & Gypsum Comb.)	severe itching; thirst; bleeding lesion
* p. 55	*Kuei-chih-chia-huang-chi-tang* (Cinnamon & Astragalus Comb.)	chronic

HICCOUGHS (eructation)

p. 407	*Ting-hsiang-shih-ti-tang* (Clove & Kaki Comb.)	if chill, white tongue coat; weak constitution
p. 374	*Chu-pi-chu-ju-tang* (Aurantium & Bamboo Comb.)	if heat (internal) conformation weak constitution tight chest, constipation dry tongue, LOUD voice

	Formula	Differentiation
* p. 212	*Ping-wei-san* (Magnolia & Ginger Formula) or	
* p. 105	*Pan-hsia-hsieh-hsin-tang* (Pinellia Comb.)	
* p. 295	*Jen-sheng-tang* (Ginseng & Ginger Comb.) plus cloves 2-6 gm cinnamon 2-6 gm aconite ½-1 gm	yang *xu*
* p. 110	*Sheng-chiang-hsieh-hsin-tang* (Pinellia & Ginger Comb.) or Pinellia Combination	food accumulation w̄ powerful hiccoughs; foul breath alternating diarrhea/constipation
* p. 366	*An-chung-san* (Cardamon & Fennel Formula)	severe abdominal gas/pain
p. 551	*Er-chen-tang* (Citrus & Pinellia Comb.) plus poncirus (*chih-shih*) bamboo stem *shen-chu* crataegus malt	cold, water toxicity in stomach nausea with hiccoughs sputum, chest,distress, cough add ginger bamboo sap lindera saussurea
p. 90	*Chu-ju-wen-tan-tang* (Bamboo & Ginseng Comb.)	stagnant heat in chest and stomach febrile diseases; hot sputum flushed; hypertensive
p. 154	*Tiao-wei-cheng-chi-tang* (Rhubarb & Mirabilitum Comb.)	strong patient w̄ constipation
* p. 212	*Ping-wei-san* (Magnolia & Ginger Formula)	excessive food intake w̄ hiccoughs food stagnation; foul breath
**** p. 404	*Shih-ti-tang* (Kaki Combination)	COLD stomach, submerged pulse cold limbs
**** p. 374	*Chu-pi-chu-ju-tang* (Aurantium & Bamboo Comb.)	HOT stomach, weaker patient; chest obstructed feeling; flushing up
p. 407	*Ting-hsiang-shih-ti-tang* (Clove & Kaki Combination)	more severe stomach weakness; *xu* pt yang *xu;* white tongue coat

p. 287	*Fu-tzu-li-chung-tang* (Aconite, Ginseng, & Ginger Comb.)	severe spleen/stomach yang *xu* severe diarrhea/abd. pain
* p. 313	*Szu-ni-tang* (Aconite & G. L. Combination)	superficial fever, internal chill spleen yang *xu*

BELCHING

* p. 110	*Sheng-chiang-hsieh-hsin-tang* (Pinellia & Ginger Combination)	stomach *qi xu*; food stagnation diarrhea (*shao* yang)
*** p. 105	*Pan-hsia-hsieh-hsin-tang* (Pinellia Combination)	food stagnation (cold); spleen *qi* xu restless; diarrhea anorexia
* p. 384	*Hsuan-fu-hua-tai-che-shih-tang* (Inula & Hematite Combination)	yin *xu* heat-weakness; stagnant stomach water

INSOMNIA

Heart/Spleen *Qi Xu*

* p. 425	Ginseng & Longan Comb. (*Kuei-pi-tang*) or	poor appetite poor memory palpitations pale face exhaustion no taste to food/drink T- thin pale P- knotted, choppy, irregular obstructed
p. 275	Astragalus & Zizyphus Comb. (*Yang-hsin-tang*)	

Yin Exhausted & Fire Flaring (Yin *Xu*)
=Heart and Kidney not – communicating
=Ki yin *xu* w̄ hyperactive heart

p. 97	Coptis & Gelatin Comb. (*Huang-lien-ah-chiao-tang*) most severe heat and/or	strong pt irritable dizziness/tinnitus low back pain dry mouth nocturnal emissions

p. 343 Cinnabar Formula
(*Chu-sha-an-shen-wan*)
severe irritability

T- red
P- thin but fast

* p. 270 Ginseng & Zizyphus Formula
(*Tien-wang-pu-hsin-tan*)™
weaker patient

exhaustion due to excessive mental work, studies

Heart/Gallbladder *Qi* Weakness (all stress conditions attack gallbladder vessel)

* p. 355 Zizyphus Combination
(*Suan-tsao-jen-tang*)
esp. if night sweats

indecision/lack of courage
panicky; irritable & hyperfunction;
easily astonished
always afraid
many dreams
T- pale
P- thin, tight

* p. 425 Ginseng & Longan Comb.
(*Kuei-pi-tang*)
esp. if poor appetite

or

Ginseng and Polygala Formula
(*An-shen-ting-chih-wan*)

ginseng	6 gm
hoelen/*fu-ling*	6 gm
hoelen centers/*fu-shen*	6 gm
polygala	6 gm
dragon bone	3 gm
acorus	3 gm

Stomach & Middle *Jiao* without Harmony

p. 114 Bamboo & Hoelen Combination
(*Wen-tan-tang*)

sputum w̄ fire accumulation (phlegm)
thirst
dizziness
bitter taste
chest distress
difficult urination/defecation
weak pt
nightmares/neurotic hyper-sensitive
gastric distress
spont./night sweats

	Formula	Indication
p. 212	Citrus & Crataegus Formula (*Pao-ho-wan*)	food accumulation gastric distress poor digestion/belching T- yellow, greasy coat P- full, smooth, fast slippery

Heart/Kidney Disharmony/Yin *Xu*

	Formula	Indication
* p. 245	Rehmannia 6 Formula (*Liu-wei-ti-huang-wan*)	if low back pain predominates nocturnal emission
* p. 175	Coptis & Scute Combination (*Huang-lien-chieh-tu-tang*)	irritable, anxious w̄ flushing severe hypertensive or severe menopausal symptoms
* p. 190	Coptis & Rhubarb Combination	
* p. 103	Pinellia & Licorice Combination (*Kan-tsao-hsieh-hsin-tang*)	full abdomen/many dreams borborygmus gastric prolapse dry heaves
p. 114	Bamboo & Hoelen Combination (*Wen-tan-tang*)	weak after passing stool easily frightened
	Chia-wei-wen-tan-tang =Bamboo & Hoelen plus zizyphus 5 gm coptis 1 gm	dyspnea w̄ anorexia
p. 90	Bamboo & Ginseng Combination (*Chu-ju-wen-tan-tang*)	insomnia during common cold or pneumonia or flu w̄ stagnant heat in chest
* p. 425	Ginseng & Longan Combination (*Kuei-pi-tang*)	anemia w̄ poor memory palpitations, esp. in elderly
	and/or	
* p. 343	Bupleurum Formula (*I-kan-san*)	emotional distress, panic
* p. 355	Zizyphus Combination (*Suan-tsao-jen-tang*)	exhausted with spontaneous sweating
p. 192	Scute Three Herb Combination (*San-wu-huang-chin-tang*)	female yin *xu* non-responsive to other formulas extreme thirst/dry mouth irritability

* p. 164	Lotus Seed Combination (*Ching-hsin-lien-tzu-yin*)	weak pt w̄ dysuria or nocturnal emissions or urethritis
* p. 472	Polyporus Combination (*Chu-ling-tang*)	thirst & dysuria
* p. 128	Major Bupleurum Combination (*Ta-chai-hu-tang*) - strong pt	nightly abdominal fullness
	or	
* p. 340	Bupleurum & Dragon Bone Comb. (*Chai-hu-chia-lung-ku-mu-li-tang*) - weak pt	
* p. 85	Bupleurum, Cinnamon, & Ginger Comb. (*Chai-hu-kuei-chih-kan-chiang-tang*)	extreme weakness/dyspnea dry mouth, many dreams cold limbs
* p. 108	Peony & Licorice Combination (*Shao-yao-kan-tsao-tang*)	infant night crying/colic
	or	
* p. 291	Minor Cinnamon & Peony Comb. (*Hsiao-chien-chung-tang*)	weak children
	or	
* p. 343	Bupleurum Formula (*I-kan-san*)	if extremely irritable
* p. 425	Ginseng & Longan Combination (*Kuei-pi-tang*)	anemia w̄ insomnia
* p. 262	Ginseng & Tang-kuei 10 Comb. (*Shih-chuan-ta-pu-tang*)	post-surgical weakness
	or	
* p. 239	Ginseng Nutritive Combination (*Jen-sheng-yang-yung-tang*)	cold extremities, poor appetite
* p. 351	Cinnamon & Dragon Bone Comb. (*Kuei-chih-chia-lung-ku-mu-li-tang*)	insomnia w̄ heart palpitations
* p. 87	Bupleurum & Peony Formula (*Chia-wei-hsiao-yao-san*)	insomnia w̄ menstrual dysfunction or menopausal symptoms
* p. 355	Zizyphus Combination (*Suan-tsao-jen-tang*)	insomnia w̄ chronic illness dehydration night sweats

LEUKORRHEA

	Formula	Indications
* p. 181	Gentiana Combination (*Lung-tan-hsieh-kan-tang*)	strong patient hot, yellow discharge pain
* p. 618	Tang-kuei and Eight Herb Formula (*Pa-wei-tai-hsia-fang*) (or Tang-kuei & Peony Formula)	weaker patient chronic white discharge abdominal laxity; anemia
* p. 164	Lotus Seed Combination (*Ching-hsin-lien-tzu-yin*)	very weak (ki *xu*) pt watery discharge anorexia; dry, bitter mouth nervousness
* p. 87	Bupleurum & Peony Formula (*Chia-wei-hsiao-yao-san*)	menopausal syndrome
* p. 588	Tang-kuei & Evodia Combination (*Wen-ching-tang*)	chills at waist; watery discharge
* p. 295	Ginseng & Ginger Combination (*Jen-sheng-tang*)	spleen/stomach yang *xu* poor appetite, diarrhea
	with	
* p. 242	Major Six Herb Combination (*Liu-chun-tzu-tang*)	
	or	
* p. 130	Tang-kuei & Magnolia Formula (*Wu-chi-san*)	spleen/stomach yang *xu*

LIVER DISORDERS

most commonly used

	Formula	Indications
p. 128	Major Bupleurum Combination (*Ta-chai-hu-tang*)	Pain in liver area; freq. constipation strong pt
p. 91	Minor Bupleurum Comb. (*Hsiao-chai-hu-tang*)	slightly weaker; no constipation
p. 108	Peony & Licorice Comb. (*Shao-yao-kan-tsao-tang*)	gallstone colic, strong pt
p. 117	Bupleurum & Cinnamon Comb. (*Chai-hu-kuei-chih-tang*)	gallstone colic, weaker pt spontaneous sweating frequent colds

p. 519	Capillaris Combination (*Yin-chen-hao-tang*)	icterus; jaundice with fever and constipation
p. 521	Capillaris & Hoelen 5 Comb.	combined liver & kidney disease

MASTITIS

* p. 624	Bupleurum & Schizonepeta Comb. (*Shih-wei-pai-tu-tang*)	internal heat irritability hypersensitivity, possibly suppuration
* p. 632	Lithospermum & Oyster Shell Comb. (*Tzu-ken-mu-li-tang*)	chronic benign mastitis anemia
* p. 402	Tang-kuei 16 Herb Combination (*Shih-liu-wei-liu-chi-yin*)	breast swelling and chronic fibrocystic disease

MENOPAUSE

* p. 87	Bupleurum & Peony Combination (*Chia-wei-hsiao-yao-san*)	emotional instability many complaints, nagging low back pain flushing/yin *xu* heat menstrual irregularity
* p. 343	Bupleurum Formula (*I-kan-san*)	very unstable emotions terror, panic
* p. 395	Pinellia & Magnolia Comb. (*Pan-hsia-hou-pu-tang*)	hysteria something "stuck in the throat" sleep disorders
* p. 425	Ginseng & Longan Combination (*Kuei-pi-tang*)	palpitations poor memory
p. 114	Bamboo & Hoelen Combination (*Wen-tan-tang*)	easily frightened insomnia nightmares spont. sweating
* p. 351	Cinnamon & Dragon Bone Comb. (*Kuei-chih-chia-lung-ku-mu-li-tang*)	weak and cold nervous palpitations
* p. 175	Coptis & Scute Combination (*Huang-lien-chieh-tu-tang*)	flushed, normal bowels insomnia

p. 394	Tang-kuei & Cyperus Comb. (*Nu-shen-san*)	flushing anxiety/depression low back pain
* p. 117	Bupleurum & Cinnamon Comb. (*Chai-hu-kuei-chih-tang*)	yawning headaches/insomnia abdominal/chest distress
* p. 340	Bupleurum & Dragon Bone Comb. (*Chai-hu-chia-lung-ku-mu-li-tang*)	nervous constipated hypertensive umbilical palpitation

MENTAL DISTRESS

Seven Emotions

Excessive Pleasure Injures the Heart and Loosens *Qi*

p. 190	Coptis & Rhubarb Combination (*San-huang-hsieh-hsin-tang*)	inappropriate laughter (when discussing symptoms) w̄ constipation
p. 175	Coptis & Scute Combination (*Huang-lien-chieh-tu-tang*)	without constipation

Nourishing the Heart & Spleen

p. 425	Ginseng & Longan Combination (*Kuei-pi-tang*)	poor memory; excessive mental activity- students

Anger Injures the Liver Producing Flushing Up of *Qi*

p. 343	Bupleurum Formula (*I-kan-san*)	severe anger w̄ shaking, palsy
p. 114	Bamboo & Hoelen Combination (*Wen-tan-tang*)	GI weakness w̄ insomnia
p. 87	Bupleurum & Peony Formula (*Chia-wei-hsiao-yao-san*)	menopausal irritability
p. 91	Minor Bupleurum Combination (*Hsiao-chai-hu-tang*)	more severe chest distress

Fear/Fright Injures Blood Affecting the Kidneys Producing Sexual Weakness

p. 250	Rehmannia 8 Formula (*Pa-wei-ti-huang-wan*)	weak, elderly, chronic yang *xu* cold and weak lower extremities

p. 245	Rehmannia 6 Formula (*Liu-wei-ti-huang-wan*)	weak *yin xu,* night sweats low back pain
p. 359	Lotus Stamen Formula (*Chin-sou-ku-ching-wan*)	nocturnal emission; low back pain
p. 270	Ginseng & Zizyphus Formula (*Tien-wang-pu-hsin -tan*)	mental exhaustion; spermatorrhea poor memory
p. 237	Lycium Formula (*Huan-shao-tan*)	sexual weakness in young persons (under age 40)

Sorrow/Anxiety Injures the Lungs; Obstructs and Injures *Qi*

p. 548	Platycodon & Fritillary Comb. (*Ching-fei-tang*)	profuse, thick, tenacious sputum
p. 537	Ophiopogon Combination (*Mai-men-tung-tang*)	red face, dry harsh cough
p. 359	Lotus Stamen Formula (*Chin-sou-ku-ching-wan*)	kidney weakness secondary to lung disorder
p. 253	Lily Combination (*Pai-ho-ku-chin-tang*)	lung yin deficiency dry cough, night sweats

Excessive Cognition, Meditation, Pensiveness Injures the Spleen and Coagulates *Qi*

p. 516	Hoelen 5 Herb Formula (*Wu-ling-san*)	thirst, dysuria, headache
p. 260	Ginseng & Atractylodes Comb. (*Sheng-ling-pai-chu-san*)	severe weakness, anorexia diarrhea

NECK-SHOULDER STIFFNESS

* p. 122	*Ko-ken-huang-lien-huang-chin-tang* (Pueraria, Coptis, & Scute Comb.)	with diarrhea
* p. 119	*Fang-feng-tung-sheng-san* (Siler & Platycodon Formula)	with constipation, yang *shi* liver excess but no chest pain overeating, hypertension
* p. 128	*Ta-chai-hu-tang* (Major Bupleurum Combination)	right side (from liver) w gallstones, obesity, constipation, hypertension
* p. 91	*Hsiao-chai-hu-tang* (Minor Bupleurum Combination)	weak pt chest distress

* p. 340	*Chai-hu-chia-lung-ku-mu-li-tang* (Bupleurum & Dragon Bone Comb.)	palpitations/dizziness/hypertension
* p. 117	*Chai-hu-kuei-chih-tang* (Bupleurum & Cinnamon Comb.)	soft abdomen/umbilical palpitation weak pulse
* p. 87	*Chia-wei-hsiao-yao-san* (Bupleurum & Peony Formula)	menstrual/menopause disorder
* p. 190	*San-huang-hsieh-hsin-tang* (Coptis & Rhubarb Comb.)	flushing, dizzy, hypertension constipation
* p. 175	*Huang-lien-chieh-tu-tang* (Coptis & Scute Comb.)	above w̄ no constipation
* p. 585	*Tang-kuei-shao-yao-san* (Tang-kuei & Peony Comb.)	chronic kidney disease; low back pain nocturia w̄ anemia; female
* p. 250	Rehmannia 8 Formula (*Pa-wei-ti-huang-wan*)	chronic kidney disease; weak lower limbs, nocturia, elderly female
p. 411	*Yen-nien-pan-hsia-tang* (Evodia & Pinellia Comb.)	left shoulder w̄ GI inflammation or pancreatitis

***Tai* Yang**

* p. 51	*Ko-ken-tang* (Pueraria Combination)	headache, no sweating, tight jaw general ache; strong pt
* p. 63	*Kuei-chih-tang* (Cinnamon Combination)	headache; sweating; weak pt general ache

better effect: substitute Hoelen & Atractylodes for Cinnamon

hoelen	4 gm
atractylodes	4 gm
ginger	4 gm
peony	4 gm
licorice	2 gm
jujube	4 gm

* p. 278	*Chen-wu-tang* (Vitality Combination)	yang *xu*, severely chilled, weak
* p. 295	*Jen-sheng-tang* (Ginseng & Ginger Comb.)	yang *xu*, mildly chilled, weak
* p. 119	*Fang-feng-tung-sheng-san* (Siler & Platycodon Formula)	obesity w̄ constipation; *shi* pt

* p. 477	*Fang-chi-huang-chi-tang* (Stephania & Astragalus Comb.)	obesity w̄ spont. sweating; weak extremities
* p. 325	*Wu-chu-yu-tang* (Evodia Combination)	severe headaches or migraines that provoke vomiting
* p. 961	*Pan-hsia-pai-chu-tien-ma tang* (Pinellia & Gastrodia Comb.)	dizziness/headache/vomiting
* p. 409	*Wu-yao-shun-chi-san* (Lindera Formula)	post stroke stiffness
* p. 395	*Pan-hsia-hou-pu-tang* (Pinellia & Magnolia Comb.)	neurotic or shock induced shoulder stiffness insomnia, globus hystericus
		due to internal blood stagnation
* p. 87	*Chia-wei-hsiao-yao-san* (Bupleurum & Peony Formula)	dizziness w̄ flushing (*qi* rising) back pain; menstrual irregularity
* p. 585	*Tang-kuei-shao-yao-san* (Tang-kuei & Peony Comb.)	heavy head; weak constitution yang *xu;* back pain
* p. 435	*Tao-ho-cheng-chi-tang* (Persica & Rhubarb Comb.)	amenorrhea w̄ constipation; *shi* but cold feet
* p. 423	*Kuei-chih-fu-ling-wan* (Cinnamon & Hoelen Formula)	amenorrhea w̄ no constipation; *xu*
p. 437	*Ti-tang-tang* (Rhubarb and Leech Comb.) if hard on stomach use:	chronic amenorrhea; unresponsive menstrual disorders; purple lips/tongue
* p. 585	*Tang-kuei-shao-yao-san* (Tang-kuei & Peony Formula) 50:50	
* p. 423	*Kuei-chih-fu-ling-wan* (Cinnamon & Hoelen Formula)	
* p. 105	*Pan-hsia-hsieh-hsin-tang* (Pinellia Combination)	gastric ulcer/prolapse hyperchlorhydria
* p. 242	*Liu-chun-tzu-tang* (Major 6 Herb Combination)	w̄ abdominal fullness after eating weak pt
* p. 119	*Fang-feng-tung-sheng-san* (Siler & Platycodon Formula)	strong pt constipated

NEURALGIA

Page	Formula	Indication
		wind-damp
p. 38	*Chiu-wei-chiang-huo-tang* (Chianghuo Combination)	strong pt; superficial fever no sweating, stiff shoulders general ache
		due to wind-chill
* p. 51	Pueraria Combination (*Ko-ken-tang*)	strong pt; stiff shoulders general ache; difficult limb movement no sweating
* p. 76	Mahuang Combination (*Ma-huang-tang*)	severe muscle pain w̄/high fever
* p. 63	Cinnamon Combination (*Kuei-chih-tang*)	neuralgia w̄ spontaneous sweating weak pt; fever general ache
p. 145	Major Rhubarb Combination (*Ta-cheng-chi-tang*)	strong stomach w̄ constipation neuralgia
p. 170	Rhinoceros & Rehmannia Comb. (*Hsi-chiao-ti-huang-tang*)	*ying qi* injured by heat unconsciousness or delirium/convulsions whole body hot/red blood in stool, epistaxis
* p. 551	Citrus & Pinellia Combination (*Erh-chen-tang*)	internal phlegm obstruction convulsed extremities, headache neck stiffness weak St/Sp
		neuralgia due to blood weakness **neck/back stiff**
* p. 239	Ginseng Nutritive Combination (*Jen-sheng-yang-yung-tang*)	dizziness, insomnia, restless weak, tight pulse
* p. 425	Ginseng & Longan Combination (*Kuei-pi-tang*)	
* p. 343	Bupleurum Formula (*I-kan-san*)	neurotic hypersensitivity, bruxism

p. 97	Coptis & Gelatin Combination (*Huang-lien-ah-chiao-tang*)	stiff, slow movement irritable, anxious

NUMBNESS/JOINT PAIN (*Ma Bi Zheng*)

WIND/WANDERING NUMBNESS — **Polyarthritis**

* p. 489	Coix Combination (*I-yi-jen-tang*)	arthralgia with febrile polyrheumatism
* p. 450	Cinnamon & Anemarrhena Comb. (*Kuei-chih-shao-yao-chih-mu-tang*)	chronic arthralgia edema feet; low back pain ki yin *xu* labored breathing
p. 457	Major Siler Combination (*Ta-fang-feng-tang*)	rheumatoid arthritis esp. knee; partial paralysis
* p. 459	Tuhuo & Vaeicum Combination (*Tu-huo-chi-sheng-tang*)	chronic arthritis esp. sciatica/low back numb, chill legs ki *qi xu*

COLD/FIXED NUMBNESS

* p. 314	Aconite & G. L. Combination	severe arthralgia
p. 327	Wu-tou & Cinnamon Combination (*Wu-tou-kuei-chih-tang*)	severe pain/paralysis abdominal pain
* p. 304	Cinnamon & Atractylodes Comb. (*Kuei-chih-chia-ling-chu-fu-tang*)	milder fixed arthritis, arthralgia

DAMP/HEAVY NUMBNESS

* p. 489	Coix Combination plus stephania *chianghuo* or 6 gm stephania alone siler	deformed joints; muscular atrophy
p. 444	Chianghuo & Tumeric Comb.	

DAMP-HEAT NUMBNESS in Lower *Jiao* — reddish, burning urine

* p. 506	Tang-kuei & Anemarrhena Comb. (*Tang-kuei-nien-tung-tang*)	arthralgia w̄ swelling; dermatitis chill

* p. 521	Capillaris & Hoelen Formula (*Yin-chen-wu-ling-san*)	arthralgia/swelling in knees; obese/edema/sweating/heaviness weak pt

HEAT NUMBNESS **Rheumatoid Arthritis**

* p. 450	Cinnamon & Anemarrhena Comb. (*Kuei-chih-shao-yao-chih-mu-tang*)	red, swollen, painful joints
* p. 523	Atractylodes Combination (*Yueh-pi-chia-chu-tang*)	legs, feet; internal heat/sweat edema; oliguria; constipation

NUTRITIVE–TONIFYING

* p. 239	*Jen-sheng-yang-yung-tang* (Ginseng Nutritive Comb.)	weak vitality, anemia general debility sweating (*qi xu*)
* p. 262	*Shih-chuan-ta-pu-tang* (Ginseng & Tang-kuei 10 Comb.)	weak vitality, anemia no sweating/dryness (blood *xu*)
* p. 264	*Szu-chun-tzu-tang* (Major 4 Herb Combination)	weak digestion; no cold limbs dry throat/voice (spleen *qi xu*)
* p. 242	*Liu-chun-tzu-tang* (Major 6 Herb Combination)	Weak digestion; cold limbs sputum; moist throat (spleen and kidney yang *xu*)

PAIN

Shoulder/Neck

p. 128	Major Bupleurum Combination (*Ta-chai-hu-tang*)	strong pt w̄ heat "Managers' disease" chest distress constipation hypertension gallstones/gout
p. 119	Siler & Platycodon Formula (*Fang-feng-tung-sheng-san*)	strong pt w̄ heat hypertension w̄ obesity, constipation no chest distress

Page	Formulation	Differentiation
p. 340	Bupleurum & Dragon Bone Comb. (*Chai-hu-chia-lung-ku-mu-li-tang*)	less strong w̄ mild heat nervous constitution palpitation
p. 435	Persica & Rhubarb Comb. (*Tao-ho-cheng-chi-tang*)	strong w̄ constipation stagnant blood (abdominal)
p. 51	Pueraria Combination (*Ko-ken-tang*)	strong pt w̄ cold shoulder pain after flu whiplash
p. 91	Minor Bupleurum Comb. (*Hsiao-chai-hu-tang*)	slightly weak w̄ chest distress/shoulder stiff white tongue coating
p. 105	Pinellia Combination (*Pan-hsia-hsieh-hsin-tang*)	slightly weak w̄ GI distress appetite poor stomach "water toxin" dry heaves hangover shoulder stiffness
p. 242	Major Six Herb Combination (*Liu-chun-tzu-tang*)	slightly weak w̄ cold easily fatigued- *qi xu* extremities cold/GI distress
p. 395	Pinellia & Magnolia Comb. (*Pan-hsia-hou-pu-tang*)	weak and cold pt stagnant *qi*- "stuck in throat" epigastric "water accumulation"
p. 87	Bupleurum & Peony Formula (*Chia-wei-hsiao-yao-san*)	weak & slight heat menopausal chest distress/stagnant blood
p. 585	Tang-kuei & Peony Formula (*Tang-kuei-shao-yao-san*)	weak & cold pt anemia, esp. female infertility; some GI side effects nausea, diarrhea
p. 561	Pinellia & Gastrodia Comb. (*Pan-hsia-pai-chu-tien-ma-tang*)	weak & cold- hypotensive anemia w̄ dizziness chronic headaches; tired after eating
p. 85	Bupleurum, Cinnamon, & Ginger Combination (*Chai-hu-kuei-chih-kan-chiang-tang*)	very weak & cold slight chest distress insomnia; cold extremities spont. sweating

Rheumatic Pain

"Wandering or 'Hot' *bi*"

Page	Formula	Indication
p. 108	Peony & Licorice Combination (*Shao-yao-kan-tsao-tang*)	acute muscle pain/spasm gall/kidney stone colic dysmenorrhea
p. 506	Tang-kuei & Anemarrhena Comb. (*Tang-kuei-nien-tung-tang*)	chronic: all types whole body pain meridian/muscle spasm/joint 'rheumatoid arthritis'
p. 429	Clematis & Stephania Comb. (*Shu-ching-huo-hsieh-tang*)	sciatica; muscular rheumatism esp. w̄ stagnant blood
p. 454	Clematis & Carthamus Formula (*Shu-chin-li-an-san*)	acute/chronic rheumatoid arthritis esp. knees
p. 293	Atractylodes Combination (*Huang-chi-chien-chung-tang*)	edema, thirst, heat strong pt Reiter's Syndrome severe conjunctivitis dysuria rheumatoid arthritis
p. 489	Coix Combination (*I-yi-jen-tang*)	subclinical arthritis "cervical-brachial osteoarthritis" pain down arm strong pt w̄ pain/swelling/ fever
p. 66	Mahuang & Coix Comb. (*Ma-hsing-i-kan-tang*)	acute episode rheumatism or arthritis
p. 423	Cinnamon & Hoelen Formula (*Kuei-chih-fu-ling-wan*)	slightly weak w̄ chill stagnant blood–chronic pain post-traumatic rheumatism
p. 51	Pueraria Combination (*Ko-ken-tang*)	slightly weak w̄ chill no inflammatory heat acute episode osteo-arthritis
p. 302	Cinnamon & Aconite Comb. (*Kuei-chih-chia-fu-tzu-tang*) if not effective, use	weak w̄ cold chronic pain
p. 429	Clematis & Stephania Comb.	
p. 319	Tang-kuei, Evodia, & Ginger Comb. (*Tang-kuei-szu-ni-chia-wu-chu-yu-sheng-chiang-tang*)	weak w̄ cold poor circulation

Page	Formula	Differentiation
p. 130	Tang-kuei & Magnolia Formula (*Wu-chi-san*)	weak w̄ severe chill chronic severe pain
p. 250	Rehmannia 8 Formula (*Pa-wei-ti-huang-wan*) if stomach weak, or upsets stomach, use:	weak w̄ chill low back pain weak lower limbs chronic pain in elderly esp. diabetes w̄ thirst abnormal urination
p. 245	Rehmannia 6 Formula (*Liu-wei-ti-huang-wan*)	

Osteo-arthritis

Page	Formula	Differentiation
p. 523	Atractylodes Combination (*Yueh-pi-chia-chu-tang*)	strong pt w̄ systemic heat acute fever, thirst sweating & edema
p. 489	Coix Combination (*I-yi-jen-tang*)	strong pt subacute joint swelling
p. 66	Mahuang & Coix Combination (*Ma-hsing-i-kan-tang*)	acute stage polyarthritis w̄ extremity swelling, heat
p. 51	Pueraria Combination (*Ko-ken-tang*)	acute stage w̄ slight swelling
p. 302	Cinnamon & Aconite Comb. (*Kuei-chih-chia-fu-tzu-tang*)	weak w̄ chill chronic fixed pain

Headache

Page	Formula	Differentiation
p. 128	Major Bupleurum Comb. (*Ta-chai-hu-tang*)	strong pt w̄ heat hypertensive chest distress gout, gallstones
p. 340	Bupleurum & Dragon Bone Comb. (*Chai-hu-chia-lung-ku-mu-li-tang*)	strong pt w̄ heat anxious, irritable insomnia, palpitations
p. 175	Coptis & Scute Comb. (*Huang-lien-chieh-tu-tang*)	less strong w̄ heat *qi* rising/flushed face epistaxis, hypertension heavy head menopausal alcoholic insomnia

if CHRONIC hypertensive, use 50:50 with Bupleurum & Dragon Bone Combination

p. 435	Persica & Rhubarb Comb. (*Tao-ho-cheng-chi-tang*)	strong pt w̄ neat stagnant blood acute abdominal pain headaches before menses
p. 50	Pueraria & Magnolia Comb. (*Ko-ken-chia-hsin-i-chuan-chiung*)	strong pt w̄ heat w̄ nasal congestion
p. 51	Pueraria Combination (*Ko-ken-tang*)	strong pt w̄ chill acute stage colds/fever
p. 516	Hoelen 5 Herb Formula (*Wu-ling-san*)	slightly strong w̄ slight heat vascular migraine headaches
p. 386	Gambir Formula (*Kou-teng-san*)	weak pt w̄ heat hypertensive morning headahce
p. 325	Evodia Combination (*Wu-chu-yu-tang*)	weak w̄ cold cold extremities weak GI chronic headache, migraines w̄/vomiting
p. 319	Tang-kuei, Evodia, & Ginger Comb. (*Tang-kuei-szu-ni-chia-wu-chu-yu-sheng-chiang-tang*)	weak w̄ cold cold extremities w̄/cyanosis long term administration post-surgery
p. 343	Bupleurum Formula (*I-kan-san*)	weak pt w̄ heat irritable, nervous insomnia childrens' anger/tantrums
p. 87	Bupleurum & Peony Formula (*Chia-wei-hsiao-yao-san*)	weak pt w̄ heat menopausal
p. 561	Pinellia & Gastrodia Comb. (*Pan-hsia-pai-chu-tien-ma-tang*)	weak pt w̄ cold stomach distress; tired after eating hypotension dizziness

Back Pain

p. 435	Persica & Rhubarb Comb. (*Tao-ho-cheng-chi-tang*)	strong pt w̄ heat stagnant blood abdomen traumatic injury to back constipation, menstrual disorders

Page	Formula	Differentiation
p. 423	Cinnamon & Hoelen Formula (*Kuei-chih-fu-ling-wan*)	slightly weak w̄ chills flushing chronic back pain injury female stagnant blood menstrual disorders
p. 51	Pueraria Combination (*Ko-ken-tang*)	strong pt w̄ chills fever w̄ acute low back pain
p. 429	Clematis & Stephania Combination (*Shu-ching-huo-hsieh-tang*) if SEVERE use 50:50 w̄ Cinnamon & Hoelen Formula	slightly weak w̄ severe back pain stagnant blood extruded disc/sciatica minimal relief from acupuncture
p. 319	Tang-kuei, Evodia, & Ginger Comb. (*Tang-kuei-szu-ni-chia-wu chu-yu-sheng-chiang-tang*)	weak w̄ chills cold extremities
p. 130	Tang-kuei & Magnolia Formula (*Wu-chi-san*)	weak w̄ chills cold aggravates pain
p. 585	Tang-kuei & Peony Formula (*Tang-kuei-shao-yao-san*)	weak w̄ chills back pain during/after pregnancy anemia, kidney disease
p. 250	Rehmannia 8 Formula (*Pa-wei-ti-huang-wan*)	weak w̄ chills esp. elderly low back; weak legs scoliosis osteoporosis
p. 262	Ginseng & Tang-kuei 10 Comb. (*Shih-chuan-ta-pu-tang*)	severely weak; after surgery long illnesses myasthenia gravis
p. 255	Ginseng & Astragalus Combination (*Pu-chung-i-chi-tang*)	after surgery weak, poor GI function shortness of breath, anorexia

Neuritis

Page	Formula	Differentiation
p. 119	Siler & Platycodon Formula (*Fang-feng-tung-sheng-san*)	strong pt w̄ heat obese hypertensive history of stroke chronic neuritis

Page	Formula	Indication
p. 435	Persica & Rhubarb Combination (*Tao-ho-cheng-chi-tang*)	strong pt w̄ heat female back neuritis due to stagnant blood injury neuritis
p. 423	Cinnamon & Hoelen Formula (*Kuei-chih-fu-ling-wan*)	slightly weak, chilled stagnant blood thin, pale, left abdominal stagnancy
p. 51	Pueraria Combination (*Ko-ken-tang*)	strong pt, w̄ chill all neuralgias above the waist trigeminal neuralgia (w̄/aconite, atractylodes)
p. 516	Hoelen 5 Herb Formula (*Wu-ling-san*)	slightly weak w̄ heat initial stage trigeminal neuralgia
p. 429	Clematis & Stephania Comb. (*Shu-ching-huo-hsieh-tang*)	slightly weak stagnant blood w̄ below waist neuralgia
p. 543	Bupleurum & Scute Comb. (*Chai-hsien-tang*)	weak pt intercostal neuralgia/pleurisy
p. 302	Cinnamon and Aconite Comb. (*Kuei-chih-chia-fu-tzu-tang*)	weak w̄ cold paralysis
p. 319	Tang-kuei, Evodia, & Ginger Comb. (*Tang-kuei-szu-ni-chia-wu-chu-yu-sheng-chiang-tang*)	weak w̄ cold cold extremities menopausal neuritis Raynaud's disease (Buerger's)
p. 130	Tang-kuei & Magnolia Formula (*Wu-chi-san*)	weak w̄ cold cold, painful chronic neuralgia
p. 295	Ginseng & Ginger Comb. (*Jen-sheng-tang*)	weak w̄ cold intercostal neuralgia w̄ GI distress, weakness
p. 250	Rehmannia 8 Formula (*Pa-wei-ti-huang-wan*)	weak w̄ chill low back pain prostatic hypertrophy elderly

Most commonly used formulas for		**Chronic Pain**
p. 51	Pueraria Combination (*Ko-ken-tang*)	shoulder/neck w̄ headahce
p. 516	Hoelen 5 Herb Formula (*Wu-ling-san*)	chronic headache (due to 'water toxin' in brain) =poor sinus/lymphatic drainage
p. 325	Evodia Combination (*Wu-chu-yu-tang*)	severe female headaches w̄ vomiting
p. 386	Gambir Formula (*Kou-teng-san*)	morning headache w̄ hypertension
p. 429	Clematis & Stephania Comb. (*Shu-ching-huo-hsieh-tang*)	chronic sciatic neuralgia
p. 319	Tang-kuei, Evodia, & Ginger Comb. (*Tang-kuei-szu-ni-chia-wu-chu-yu-sheng-chiang-tang*)	menstrual pain w̄ cold extremities
p. 130	Tang-kuei & Magnolia Formula (*Wu-chi-san*)	rheumatism w̄ cold waist, legs
p. 250	Rehmannia 8 Formula (*Pa-wei-ti-huang-wan*)	back pain, elderly w̄ weak legs cold extremities
p. 108	Peony & Licorice Combination (*Shao-yao-kan-tsao-tang*)	chronic w̄ acute episodes: menstrual, gall, urinary stone
p. 302	Cinnamon & Aconite Comb. (*Kuei-chih-chia-fu-tzu-tang*)	chronic cold pain
p. 477	Stephania & Astragalus Comb. (*Fang-chi-huang-chi-tang*)	knee & lower extremity pain
p. 87	Bupleurum & Peony Formula	menopausal
p. 585	Tang-kuei & Peony Formula	menstrual disorder in weak, anemic pt
p. 423	Cinnamon & Hoelen Formula	menstrual disorders in strong, young pt

PALPITATIONS

* p. 500	*Mu-fang-chi-tang* (Stephania & Ginseng Comb.)	valvular heart disease congestive heart failure (cardiac asthma) edema; thirst

	Formula	Indications
* p. 529	*Chih-kan-tsao-tang* (Baked Licorice Comb.)	goiter: hyperthyroidism yin *xu* heat; red tongue; dry
* p. 340	*Chai-hu-chia-lung-ku-mu-li-tang* (Bupleurum & Dragon Bone Comb.)	mild chest distress; insomnia nervousness, edema; constipation oliguria
* p. 395	Pinellia & Magnolia Comb. (*Pan-hsia-hou-pu-tang*)	neurotic palpitations (paroxysmal atrial tachycardia fear of death; foreign sensation in throat, weak GI, fatigue
* p. 117	Bupleurum, Cinnamon, & Ginger Comb. (*Chai-hu-kuei-chih-kan-chiang-tang*)	weak pt; GI weakness, neurosia arthralgia
* p. 291	*Hsiao-chien-chung-tang* (Minor Cinnamon & Peony Comb.)	surface weak (sweating) tonify middle *jiao* first

HEART *XUE XU*

	Formula	Indications
* p. 425	*Kuei-pi-tang* (Ginseng & Longan Comb.)	very weak, poor memory
* p. 355	*Suan-tsao-jen-tang* (Zizyphus Combination)	fatigue; severe insomnia

HEART YIN *XU RE*

	Formula	Indications
* p. 270	*Tien-wang-pu-hsin-tan* (Ginseng & Zizyphus Formula)	hysteria; poor memory; emotional constipation, stomatitis
* p. 114	*Wen-tan-tang* (Bamboo & Hoelen Comb.)	food stagnation; insomnia; palpitations
p. 343	Cinnabar Formula (*Chu-sha-an-shen-wan*)	irascible, nightmares, insomnia

HEART YANG *XU*

	Formula	Indications
p. 479	*Fu-ling-kan-tsao-tang* (Licorice & Hoelen Comb.)	valvular heart disease; cold limbs spont. sweating; insomnia
* p. 493	*Ling-kuei-chu-kan-tang* (Atractylodes & Hoelen Comb.)	headache, dizziness; cold feet hyperventilation

SHOCK

* p. 351 *Kuei-chih-chia-lung-ku-mu-li-tang* (Cinnamon & Dragon Bone Comb.) — neurasthenia; nervous exhaustion

PARALYSIS/ MUSCLE ATROPHY

Weak Lung Heat w̄ Heart Irritability

* p. 548 Platycodon & Fritillaria Comb. (*Ching-fei-tang*)

dry mouth-thick sputum, cough
dry skin, no sweating
reddish, hot URINE

or

* p. 532 Eriobotrya & Ophiopogon Comb. (*Ching-tsao-chiu-fei-tang*)

Heart/Spleen Weak & Injured

* p. 425 Ginseng & Longan Combination (*Kuei-pi-tang*)

Liver/Kidney Weak & Injured
stress; overwork

* p. 263 Ginseng & Tang-kuei Ten Comb. (*Shih-chuan-ta-pu-tang*) plus deer horn

myasthenia gravis
dizziness
anemia, weak, dry skin

Internal Damp-Heat

San-miao-wan

phellodendron	3 gm
Atractylodes lancea	3 gm
achyranthes	3 gm
plus	
tang-kuei	3 gm
stephania	2 gm
smilax	2 gm
tortoise shell	2 gm

body yellow, swollen
chest distention
reddish urine obstructed/pain
heat in legs

Dampness Obstructing the Diaphragm

p. 551	Citrus & Pinellia Combination (*Erh-chen-tang*)	dizziness shoulder/spine pain back & knees numb extremities paralyzed & weak spleen *qi xu*
	or	
* p. 409	Lindera Formula (*Wu-yao-shun-chi-san*)	post-stroke conditions

Stagnant Blood in Meridians w̅ Pain

* p. 433	Tang-kuei Four Combination (*Szu-wu-tang*) plus persica carthamus zedoaria	extremities numb lips/tongue bluish extremities bluish/painful
	or	
* p. 435	Persica & Rhubarb Combination (*Tao-ho-cheng-chi-tang*)	strong pt; external injury contusion

PREGNANCY TOXICITY

* p. 487	Minor Pinellia & Hoelen Comb. (*Hsiao-pan-hsia-chia-fu-ling-tang*)	nausea and vomiting first trimester
* p. 585	Tang-kuei & Peony Formula (*Tang-kuei-shao-yao-san*)	prevent miscarriage relieve low back pain

RHEUMATIC

ACUTE RHEUMATIC PAIN
Initial onset
Feng Shi: **Wind–Damp**
anti-inflammatory

* p. 76	*Ma-huang-tang* (Mahuang Combination)	acute onset polyarticular rheumatism; strong pt
* p. 70	*Ma-huang-chia-chu-tang* (Mahuang & Atractylodes Comb.)	as above w̅ edema, spontaneous sweating

	Formula	Indications
* p. 63	*Kuei-chih-tang* (Cinnamon Combination) plus aconite 1 gm atractylodes 4 gm	acute onset polyarticular rheumatism; weak pt
* p. 51	*Ko-ken-tang* (Pueraria Combination) plus aconite 1 gm atractylodes 4 gm	cervico-brachial syndrome pain/numbness/tingling radiating to arm neck & shoulder pain
* p. 523	*Yueh-pi-chia-chu-tang* (Atractylodes Combination)	multiple rheumatoid arthritis gout; Reiter's syndrome (urethritis; conjunctivitis), arthritis
* p. 489	*I-yi-jen-tang* (Coix Combination) increase/add atractylodes	febrile arthritis
* p. 298	*Kan-tsao-fu-tzu-tang* (Licorice & Aconite Comb.)	severe, acute arthritic pain unable to straighten limbs
* p. 506	*Tang-kuei-nien-tung-tang* (Tang-kuei & Anemarrhena Comb.)	heat/swelling arthritis w̄/skin lesions **gout**
* p. 423	*Kuei-chih-fu-ling-wan* (Cinnamon & Hoelen Comb.)	post-traumatic arthralgia
	or	
* p. 435	*Tao-ho-cheng-chi-tang* (Persica & Rhubarb Comb.)	as above w̄/constipation, headaches
* p. 409	*Wu-yao-shun-chi-san* (Lindera Combination)	left shoulder/whiplash, post CVA arthralgia
p. 145	*Ta-cheng-chi tang* (Major Rhubarb Comb.)	knee pain w̄ abdominal fullness constipation
	or	
* p. 128	*Ta-chai-hu-tang* (Major Bupleurum Comb.)	as above w̄/chest distress
*		**RHEUMATIC BACK PAIN**
* p. 108	*Shao-yao-kan-tsao-tang* (Peony & Licorice Comb.)	Coldness in lumbar, aching muscle spasms
p. 321	*Tang-kuei-szu-ni-tang* (Tang-kuei & Jujube Comb.)	severe pain better w̄/heat abdominal distention or cramps

also:
Shao-kan-huang-hsin-fu-tang

peony	5	gm
licorice	1.5	gm
rhubarb	1	gm
asarum	3	gm
aconite	1	gm

* p. 423	*Kuei-chih-fu-ling-wan* (Cinnamon & Hoelen Formula)	post-traumatic back pain
* p. 435	*Tao-ho-cheng-chi-tang* (Persica & Rhubarb Comb.)	as above
* p. 585	*Tang-kuei-shao-yao-san* (Tang-kuei & Peony Formula)	anemic, cold patient back pain during pregnancy

SEVERE RHEUMATIC PAIN

use aconite- if no thirst; no tongue coat
use gypsum- if severe thirst/vomit; tongue coat

* p. 298	*Kan-tsao-fu-tzu-tang* (Licorice & Aconite Comb.)	spontaneous sweating, dypsnea difficult extension/flexion no thirst
* p. 523	*Yueh-pi-chia-chu-tang* (Atractylodes Comb.)	edema; thirst, spontaneous sweat
	Wu-tou-tang mahuang 3 gm peony 3 gm astragalus 3 gm licorice 3 gm *wu-tou* ¾ gm wild aconite (very toxic)	very severe pain
p. 327	*Wu-tou-kuei-chih-tang* (Wu-tou & Cinnamon Comb.)	cold weak pt; abdominal pain
* p. 319	Tang-kuei, Evodia, & Ginger Comb.	cyanotic limbs severe pain ameliorated by heat
* p. 66	*Ma-hsing-i-kan-tang* (Mahuang & Coix Comb.)	locus of pain changes frequently
* p. 477	*Fang-chi-huang-chi-tang* (Stephania & Astragalus Comb.)	edema/sweating spont./obese/weak esp. arthralgia of knees

CHRONIC RHEUMATIC PAIN/ Arthralgia

* p. 304	*Kuei-chih-chia-ling-chu-fu-tang* (Cinnamon & Atractylodes Comb.)	post-stroke rheumatic arthralgia chills; spont. sweating
* p. 250	*Pa-wei-ti-huang-wan* (Rehmannia 8 Formula)	geriatric lumbago/sciatica
* p. 450	*Kuei-chih-shao-yao-chih-mu-tang* (Cinnamon & Anemarrhena Comb.)	vertigo, dyspnea, paresthesias muscular atrophy
p. 457	*Ta-fang-feng-tang* (Major Siler Combination)	paralysis in weak patient especially for KNEE problems

EXCESSIVE SALIVATION

* p. 516	*Wu-ling-san* (Hoelen Five Herb Formula)	initial stage stomach flu (vomiting follows ingestion of water) extreme thirst
* p. 295	*Jen-sheng-tang* (Ginseng & Ginger Comb.)	cold limbs, poor digestion, diarrhea
* p. 300	*Kan-tsao-kan-chiang-tang* (Licorice & Ginger Comb.)	elderly; weak patients with copious thin saliva, nocturia
* p. 175	*Huang-lien-chieh-tu-tang* (Coptis & Scute Combination)	strong patients; insomnia, restless internal heat w̄ salivation: thick, odor no constipation
* p. 190	*San-huang-hsieh-hsin-tang* (Coptis & Rhubarb Comb.)	if constipation
	Hsieh-wei-tang (Rhubarb and Pueraria Combination)	continuous salivation with dry lips constipation

rhubarb	1 gm
pueraria	6 gm
platycodon	3 gm
poncirus	2 gm
peucedanum	3 gm
apricot seed	3 gm
fresh ginger	4 gm

SEXUAL DYSFUNCTION

p. 361	Cinnamon & Dragon Bone Comb. (*Kuei-chih-chia-lung-ku-mu-li-tang*)	impotence due to nervous exhaustion cold, weak dandruff umbilical palpitations
p. 250	Rehmannia 8 Formula (*Pa-wei-ti-huang-wan*)	low back; weak lower limbs nocturia
p. 237	Lycium Formula (*Huan-shao-tan*)	spleen/kidney/heart weakness lack of interest loss of libido
p. 340	Bupleurum & Dragon Bone Comb. (*Chai-hu-chia-lung-ku-mu-li-tang*)	nervousness chest distress palpitations, constipation
p. 128	Major Bupleurum Combination (*Ta-chai-hu-tang*)	obese pt w̄ severe chest distress constipation
p. 585	Tang-kuei & Peony Formula (*Tang-kuei-shao-yao-san*)	frigidity anemia, fatigue frequent urination
p. 343	Bupleurum Formula (*I-kan-san*)	angry hysteria palpitations to umbilicus
p. 573	Cinnamon & Persica Combination (*Che-tsung-yin*)	vaginal pain on intercourse (dyspareunia) if w̄ bleeding- check for cervical CA
p. 319	Tang-kuei, Evodia, & Ginger Combination	vaginal pain after intercourse

SKIN DISORDERS

Anti-toxicity Formulas

p. 119	Siler & Platycodon Formula (*Fang-feng-tung-sheng-san*)	Strong pt, obese tendency prone to hypertension/CVA hair loss body odor menstrual irregularity constipation

	Formula	Indications
p. 477	Stephania & Astragalus Comb. (*Fang-chi-huang-chi-tang*)	weak pt spont. sweating; atonic musculature elderly, obese, flabby female pain in knees
(p. 82)*	Siler Combination (*Ching-shang-fang-feng-tang*) plus 10 gm coix	acne, eczema, gingivitis otitis media
	or	
p. 610	Siler & Coix Combination (*Ching-shang-fang-feng-tang-chia-i-yi-jen*)	for relapse of symptoms, add rhubarb (1-2 gm)
*** p. 609	Schizonepeta & Siler Formula (*Ching-fang-pai-tu-san*)	suppurative skin disorders w̄ chills/fever
p. 604	Astragalus & Platycodon Formula (*Chien-chin-nei-tuo-san*)	chronic suppuration in weak pt; otitis media hemorrhoids
p. 267	Tang-kuei & Astragalus Comb. (*Tang-kuei-pu-hsieh-tang*) astragalus 30 gm *tang-kuei* 6 gm	in very weak anemic pt
*** p. 624	Bupleurum & Schizonepeta Comb. (*Shih-wei-pai-tu-tang*) plus coix 10 gm	suppurative skin diseases allergic dermatitis
	or	
p. 51	Pueraria Combination plus coix 10 gm	
p. 445	Tang-kuei & Arctium Formula (*Hsiao-feng-san*)	wet (serous) eczema itching (internal heat) thirst
p. 439	Tang-kuei & Gardenia Comb. (*Wen-ching-yin*)	chronic dry skin disorders anemia- *xue xu* severe **itching** **mucous membrane** ulcers neurotic hypersensitivity flushing up of *qi* severe uterine bleeding persistent leukorrhea genital ulcers

* *Natural Healing with Chinese Herbs*

Page	Formula	Indication
p. 628	Ludwigia Formula (*Teng-hua-pai-tu-san*)	acute allergic skin eruption initial measles rash
p. 415	Musk & Catechu Formula (*Chi-li-san*)	local contusions
p. 160	Bupleurum & Rehmannia Comb. (*Chai-hu-ching-kan-tang*)	teenager acne; measles, tonsillitis pale, thin build; weak lymphadenitis
p. 48	Ginseng & Mentha Formula (*Jen-sheng-pai-tu-san*)	common cold w̄ skin rashes, carbuncle, joint pain nasal congestion
p. 631	Gleditsia Combination (*Tuo-li-hsiao-tu-yin*)	weak pt w̄ internal lymph suppuration poor wound healing purulent otitis media otorrhea
p. 604	Astragalus & Platycodon Formula (*Chien-chin-nei-tuo-san*)	if very weak
p. 619	Platycodon & Chih-shih Formula (*Pai-nung-san*) *chih-shih* 5 gm peony 5 gm platycodon 2 gm	deep infections, cellulitis pyorrhea, mastitis felon
p. 621	Platycodon & Jujube Comb. (*Pai-nung-tang*) licorice 3 gm ginger 3 gm platycodon 2 gm jujube 6 gm	cutaneous infections
p. 623	Forsythia & Laminaria Combination (*San-tsung-kuei-chien-tang*)	"hard" infections cervical lymphadenitis scrofula- TB in lymph nodes
p. 632	Lithospermum & Oyster Shell Comb. (*Tzu-ken-mu-li-tang*)	all swellings, esp. breast cancer mastitis malignant skin diseases lymphadenitis

SKIN LESIONS

"Athletes Foot"

	Formula	Differentiation
* p. 66	Mahuang & Coix Combination (*Ma-hsing-i-kan-tang*)	dry lesions
* p. 624	Bupleurum & Schizonepeta Comb. (*Shih-wei-pai-tu-tang*)	wet, purulent lesions
* p. 631	Gleditsia Combination (*Tuo-li-hsiao-tu-yin*)	if no response in 2 weeks with above formulas
p. 604	Astragalus & Platycodon Formula (*Chien-chin-nei-tuo-san*)	more profuse secretions
p. 192	Scute Three Herb Combination (*San-wu-huang-chin-tang*)	dryness, itching, heat
	Decoction of Sophora	external wash
p. 634	Lithospermum Ointment	promotes new skin growth

SKIN DISEASES

Eczema

	Formula	Differentiation
* p. 523	Atractylodes Combination (*Yueh-pi-chia-chu-tang*)	eczema w̄ profuse suppuration edema gastric fullness oliguria dry mouth/thirst
* p. 519	Capillaris Combination (*Yin-chen-hao-tang*)	w̄ GI heat/thirst constipation pressure in chest
* p. 128	Major Bupleurum Comb. (*Ta-chai-hu-tang*)	w̄ severe heat painful chest distress
* p. 119	Siler & Platycodon Formula (*Fang-feng-tung-sheng-san*) plus Major Bupleurum Comb.	w̄ hypertension obesity w̄ constipation auto-intoxication from overeating
* p. 435	Persica & Rhubarb Combination (*Tao-ho-cheng-chi-tang*)	chronic eczema in strong pt w̄ dirty, foul-smelling lesions, profuse suppuration

		w̄ itching scabs also for female flushing, headaches w̄ constipation/red skin
* p. 626	Rhubarb & Moutan Combination (*Ta-huang-mu-tan-pi-tang*) also if no results from Tang-kuei & Arctium Comb. Tang-kuei & Gardenia Comb.	specific for eczema of the back also lower right quadrant pain long term administration
* p. 183	Ginseng & Gypsum Combination (*Pai-hu-chia-jen-sheng-tang*)	severe heat, thirst, itching w̄ insomnia, irritability
	Kuei-chi-chien-chung-tang =Minor Cinnamon & Peony Comb. plus *tang-kuei* 4 gm astragalus 2 gm	severe subcutaneous inflammation
* p. 295	Ginseng & Ginger Combination (*Jen-sheng-tang*)	children's auto-intoxication epigastric fullness cold abdomen, limbs

SKIN DISEASES—DRY LESIONS

Eczema, Dermatitis, Urticaria (hives)

* p. 51	Pueraria Combination (*Ko-ken-tang*) if excess heat add gypsum 10 gm if constipation add rhubarb 1 gm	acute stage urticaria no suppuration Tx: Induce sweating to disperse surface evil
* p.. 41	Cyperus & Perilla Formula (*Hsiang-su-san*) to increase cooling effect add gardenia 2 gm	if gastric distress esp. fish poisoning allergic dermatitis detoxify blood
* p. 624	Bupleurum & Schizonepeta Comb. (*Shih-wei-pai-tu-tang*) add: forsythia 2 gm coix 10 gm	relieves food allergy dermatitis decreases penicillin sensitivity acne w̄ hypersensitive constitution esp. if chest distress chronic genital herpes

* p. 585	Tang-kuei & Peony Formula (*Tang-kuei-shao-yao-san*) plus coix 10 gm	"age spots"
* p. 610	Siler & Coix Combination (*Ching-shang-fang-feng-tang-chia-i-yi-jen*)	acne w̄ flushing up constipation oliguria, no sweating wiry pulse
* p. 607	Schizonepeta & Forsythia Comb. (*Ching-chieh-lien-chiao-tang*)	milder case esp. oily skin
* p. 445	Tang-kuei and Arctium Formula (*Hsiao-feng-san*)	"hidden blood rash" (damp-heat) internal heat in blood lymphatic septicemia dry skin abrupt, intermittent itching extreme thirst
* p. 175	Coptis & Scute Combination (*Huang-lien-chieh-tu-tang*) or	external summer-heat rash (or) internal wind-heat w̄ boils weak *wei qi* - acne/boils in strong pt
p. 170	Rhinoceros & Rehmannia Comb.	
p. 569	Mume Formula (*Wu-mei-wan*)	worm infestation of skin
* p. 624	Bupleurum & Schizonepeta Comb. (*Shih-wei-pai-tu-tang*)	if pustular
* p. 432	Tang-kuei Four Combination (*Szu-wu-tang*)	blood weak; with wind-dryness (yin *xu*) itching but no pustules dry, rough skin esp. elderly irritable; insomnia dry mouth; night sweats
* p. 386	Gambir Formula (*Kou-teng-san*)	if extreme anger
* p. 250	Rehmannia 8 Formula (*Pa-wei-ti-huang-wan*)	liver/kidney *qi xu* dirty, tired, face color spider angioma- hair loss; dry eyes dizziness low back discomfort palms/soles hot nocturnal emissions irregular menses leukorrhea

* p. 624	Bupleurum & Schizonepeta Comb. (*Shih-wei-pai-tu-tang*) add coix in acne/eczema forsythia in urticaria	acute urticaria (hives) allergic dermatitis, eczema, acne hypersensitive, nervous costal distress
* p. 445	Tang-kuei & Arctium Formula (*Hsiao-feng-san*)	if scabs/pustular in strong pt thirst w̄ worsening of symptoms in summer
* p. 439	Tang-kuei & Gardenia Comb. (*Wen-ching-yin*)	"sunlight dermatitis" scratching produces a powdery desquamation dryness/heat/redness
	add forsythia 4 gm schizonepeta 2 gm	if severe itching
p. 540	Tang-kuei & Tribulus Comb. (*Tang-kuei-yin-tzu*)	severe dryness w̄ erythema/itching desquamation often in anemic elderly/weak pt worse in winter
p. 185	Gypsum Combination (*Pai-hu-tang*) plus coptis 2 gm	intense burning/itching eczema w̄ severe thirst/ occasional chills strong pt
* p. 119	Siler & Platycodon Formula (*Fang-feng-tung-sheng-san*)	recalcitrant eczema in strong pt obese tendency constipation
* p. 128	Major Bupleurum Combination (*Ta-chai-hu tang*) plus capillaris 3 gm gardenia 4 gm	urticaria (hives) along spine often w̄ chest distress constipation
* p. 91	Minor Bupleurum Combination (*Hsiao-chai-hu-tang*)	children's urticaria allergic dermatitis (food allergy)

SKIN DISEASES–PUSTULAR LESIONS

Furuncle/Carbuncle/Boils
Erysipelas/Cellulitis

EXTERNAL FORMULAS

Tai-yi-gao™ Plaster
(Scrophularia, Angelica, and Peony Ointment)

scrophularia	momordica
angelica	asafoetida
tang-kuei	human hair ash
cinnamon	mercuric chloride
red peony	lead oxide
rhubarb	mastic
rehmannia	myrrh
	sesame oil

Gan-zhi-gao™ pine resin plaster

wash for athletes foot
Ku-sheng-tang

sophora root	6 gm
water	500 cc

INTERNAL FORMULAS to dispel pus/reduce swelling

* p. 83	Lonicera & Forsythia Formula (*Yin-chiao-san*)	initial stage inflammation (no pus)
	or	
* p. 609	Schizonepeta & Siler Formula (*Ching-fang-pai-tu-san*)	slight cellulitis
p. 189	Scute & Cimicifuga Combination (*Pu-chi-hsiao-tu-yin*)	cellulitis w pus
	or	
* p. 175	Coptis & Scute Combination (*Huang-lien-chieh-tu-tang*)	
* p. 631	Gleditsia Combination (*Tuo-li-hsiao-tu-yin*)	if tissue very hard but no pus
p. 604	Astragalus & Platycodon Formula (*Chien-chin-nei-tuo-san*)	in weak pt, with poor wound healing
	or	
p. 317	Tang-kuei, Cinnamon, & Peony Comb. (*Tang-kuei-chien-chung-tang*)	

* p. 248	Tang-kuei & Ginseng 8 Comb. (*Pa-chen-tang*)	poor healing of furuncles/eczema
	or	
* p. 245	Rehmannia Six Formula (*Liu-wei-ti-huang-wan*)	
* p. 624	Bupleurum & Schizonepeta Comb. (*Shih-wei-pai-tu-tang*)	lymphadenitis/mastitis (no swelling)
p. 619	Platycodon & Chih-shih Formula (*Pai-nung-san*)	(if w̄ swelling)
* p. 631	Gleditsia Combination	(if w̄ pus) mild
p. 604	Astragalus & Platycodon Formula (*Chien-chin-nei-tuo-san*)	chronic, slow-healing lesions weak/post-surgical pt
	or	
p. 317	Tang-kuei, Cinnamon, & Peony Comb.	
p. 622	Eriocheir & Viper Formula (*Po-chou-san*)	chronic suppuration

SNEEZING

* p. 51	*Ko-ken-tang* (Pueraria Combination)	yang strong; general ache, spasms no sweating
* p. 43	*Hsiao-ching-lung-tang* (Minor Blue Dragon Combination)	allergic rhinitis, clear runny snivel or dry cough strong pt
* p. 537	*Mai-men-tung-tang* (Ophiopogon Combination)	dryness; internal heat; weak pt

SURGICAL WOUNDS

* p. 87	Bupleurum & Peony Formula (*Chia-wei-hsiao-yao-san*)	post surgical complications from hysterectomy
**** p. 108	Peony & Licorice Combination (*Shao-yao-kan-tsao-tang*) peony 6 gm licorice 6 gm add aconite if severe pain 1 gm	relieves spasm dispels stagnant blood checks pain

* p. 177	Sweet Combination (*Kan-lu-yin*)	mouth infections relieve stagnant heat abdominal fullness flushing up general fever
**** p. 179	Cinnamon Five Herb Combination (*Kuei-chih-wu-wu-tang*) or	stomatitis, ulcerative gingivitis toothache dispels heat, internal; flushing nourishes spleen
p. 178	Forsythia & Peony Formula (*Chia-chien-liang-ke-san*)	
* p. 624	Bupleurum & Schizonepeta Comb. (*Shih-wei-pai-tu-tang*)	swelling & inflammation, heat suppuration, lymphademoma hypersensitivity
* p. 415	Musk & Catechu Formula (*Chi-li-san*)	trauma, contusions, general pain not in pregnancy

SURGERY - post gynecological

p. 583	Tang-kuei & Ginger Combination (*Sheng-hua tang*)	postpartum bleeding and abdominal pain
p. 585	*Tang-kuei-shao-yao-san* (Tang-kuei & Peony Formula)	weak, anemic pt abdominal pain

THIRST

In general:
acute- gypsum
chronic- rehmannia
ginseng
aconite

* p. 516	Hoelen 5 Herb Formula (*Wu-ling-san*) if pt vomits on drinking water	
p. 68	Mahuang & Apricot Seed Combination (*Ma-hsing-kan-shih-tang*) mahuang 4 gm apricot seed 1 gm licorice 2 gm gypsum 10 gm	severe thirst cough sweating fever acute asthma attack

p. 220	Bamboo & Gypsum Combination (*Chu-yeh-shih-kao-tang*) also for fever of unknown origir	yang *ming* disease big thirst (not alleviated by water) big fever big pulse big abdomen cough/thick sputum dry skin/night sweats insomnia
p. 185	Gypsum Combination (*Pai-hu-tang*)	if spontaneous sweating
* p.. 183	Ginseng & Gypsum Combination (*Pai-hu-chia-jen-sheng-tang*)	chronic thirst diabetic thirst chills, constipation
* p. 519	Capillaris Combination (*Yin-chen-hao-tang*)	acute hepatitis; jaundice
* p. 521	Capillaris & Hoelen Formula (*Yin-chen-wu-ling-san*)	chronic liver/ki disease hepatitis
p. 187	Anemone Combination (*Pai-tou-weng-tang*) or	enteritis w̄ internal heat diarrhea/tenesemus leading to thirst
* p. 122	Pueraria, Coptis, & Scute Comb. (*Ko-ken-huang-lien-huang-chin-tang*)	
p. 185	Gypsum Combination (*Pai-hu-tang*)	pt desires cold drinks (*tai* yang)
* p. 278	Vitality Combination (*Chen-wu-tang*)	pt desires warm drinks (yin stage)
* p. 105	Pinellia Combination (*Pan-hsia-hsieh-hsin-tang*)	white tongue coat (gypsum forbidden) water toxin in stomach infracardiac distress diarrhea
* p. 128	Major Bupleurum Comb. (*Ta-chai-hu-tang*)	yellow tongue coat strong or obese abdominal distress
p. 185	Gypsum Combination (*Pai-hu-tang*)	severe high fever; **dry heat lu/st**
* p. 183	Ginseng & Gypsum Comb. (*Pai-hu-chia-jen-sheng-tang*)	in weaker patient

* p. 537	Ophiopogon Combination (*Mai-men-tung-tang*)	if dry harsh cough
p. 194	Major Rhubarb Comb.	severe constipation high fever; delirium
* p. 245	Rehmannia 6 Formula (*Liu-wei-ti-huang-wan*)	yin weakness with **deficiency of liquid** impotence, low back pain
* p. 177	Sweet Combination (*Kan-lu-yin*)	stomatitis
* p. 260	Ginseng & Atractylodes Formula (*Sheng-ling-pai-chu-san*)	spleen weakness w̄ **damp accumulation** anorexia enteritis; full abdomen
p. 228	Atractylodes & Pueraria Formula (*Chien-shih-pai-chu-san*)	severe spleen weakness sweet taste; spasms diabetic anorexia
* p. 250	Rehmannia 8 Formula	yang fails to transform *qi* fatigue weak extremities thirst constipation
* p. 487	Minor Pinellia & Hoelen Comb. (*Hsiao-pan-hsia-chia-fu-ling-tang*) if no response use Hoelen 5	morning sickness, pernicious vomiting

THIRST IN YIN STAGE
(without desire for drink)

* p. 295	Ginseng & Ginger Combination (*Jen-sheng-tang*) = *Li-chung-tang*	*tai* yin weakness (spleen yang *xu*); water toxin st diarrhea
* p. 291	Minor Cinnamon & Peony Comb. (*Hsiao-chien-chung-tang*)	children's digestive weakness
* p. 250	Rehmannia 8 Formula	freq. urination, low back pain, weak legs
* p. 483	Alisma & Hoelen Combination (*Fu-ling-tse-hsieh-tang*)	decreased urination vomiting abdominal distention
* p. 435	Persica & Rhubarb Comb. (*Tao-ho-cheng-chi-tang*)	*jue* yin chronic blood stagnation internal heat; cold feet delirium

* p. 278	Vitality Combination (*Chen-wu-tang*)	*jue* yin general weakness black tongue coat chill, edema
* p. 313	Aconite & G.L. Combination (*Szu-ni-tang*)	severe chill sweating spont. diarrhea
p. 283	Hoelen, G.L., & Aconite Comb. (*Fu-ling-szu-ni-tang*)	extreme chill $\overline{w}$ edema
		with ABNORMAL URINATION
* p. 250	Rehmannia 8 Formula	kidney atrophy
* p. 516	Hoelen 5 Herb Formula (*Wu-ling-san*)	oliguria $\overline{w}$ edema (nephrosis)
* p. 472	Polyporus Combination (*Chu-ling-tang*)	oliguria $\overline{w}$ hematuria pain
p. 68	Mahuang & Apricot Seed Comb. (*Ma-hsing-kan-shih-tang*)	with cough and pleurisy
* p. 81	Major Blue Dragon Combination	acute onset of pneumonia

TINNITUS

* p. 493	Atractylodes & Hoelen Comb. (*Ling-kuei-chu-kan-tang*)	water flowing upward stomach water toxin dizziness
* p. 485	Hoelen Combination (*Fu-ling-yin*)	water toxin/stagnation in stomach
	or	
* p. 105	Pinellia Combination (*Pan-hsia-hsieh-hsin-tang*)	
* p. 585	Tang-kuei & Peony Formula (*Tang-kuei-shao-yao-san*)	weakness & anemia menstrual disorders nephritis
* p. 262	Tang-kuei & Ginseng 10 Comb. (*Shih-chuan-ta-pu-tang*)	severely weakened after long illness
* p. 340	Bupleurum & Dragon Bone Comb. (*Chai-hu-chia-lung-ku-mu-li-tang*)	neurotic tinnitus $\overline{w}$ anxiety

	Formula	Differentiation
* p. 250	Rehmannia 8 Formula (*Pa-wei-ti-huang-wan*)	geriatric (ki *xu*) tinnitus polyuria lumbago
* p. 128	Major Bupleurum Combination (*Ta-chai-hu-tang*)	yang rising – shoulder stiffness hypertension flushing obesity
* p. 119	Siler & Platycodon Formula (*Fang-feng-tung-sheng-san*)	obese, constipated, hypertensive
* p. 190	Coptis & Rhubarb Combination (*San-huang-hsieh-hsin-tang*) w̄ constipation	flushing w̄ insomnia: post stroke as a stroke preventive: 1-2 gm/day w̄ food
* p. 175	Coptis & Scute Combination (*Huang-lien-chieh-tu-tang*) w̄ no constipation	
* p. 91	Minor Bupleurum Combination (*Hsiao-chai-hu-tang*) (*shao yang*)=chest distress	hearing loss after a cold
* p. 41	Cyperus & Perilla Formula (*Hsiang-su-san*) (*tai yang*)	

TCM:

	Formula	Differentiation
* p. 51	Pueraria Combination (*Ko-ken-tang*) w̄ shoulder stiffness	itching internal ear wind-heat in upper heater increasing tinnitus excessive ear wax
* p. 76	*Ma-huang-tang* w̄ general ache	
* p. 83	Lonicera & Forsythia Formula (*Yin-chiao-san*)	more severe heat
* p. 160	Bupleurum & Rehmannia (*Chai-hu-ching-kan-tang*) swollen lymph glands	fire concentrated in middle heater tinnitus w̄ headache easily angered hypochondrial distress excessive sputum in throat
* p. 271	Scute Combination (*Tzu-sheng-tung-erh-tang*)	drug-induced tinnitus

* p. 250	Rehmannia 8 Formula	weakness of kidney *qi* tinnitus w̄ difficult hearing palpitations dizziness insomnia low back pain impotence

URINARY INCONTINENCE

p. 300	Licorice & Ginger Combination (*Kan-tsao-kan-chiang-tang*) licorice 4 gm ginger 2 gm	ki not receiving *qi* dizziness excess salivation no thirst incontinence on coughing also ki yang *xu* w̄ dry mouth
* p. 260	Ginseng & Atractylodes Comb. (*Sheng-ling-pai-chu-san*)	spleen *xu* weak extremities no desire to speak poor appetite diarrhea after eating
* p. 250	Rehmannia 8 Formula plus cervus (dear antler) 3 gm	kidney yang *xu* incontinence nocturia profuse urination severe cold cold extremities P- fine
* p. 245	Rehmannia 6 Formula (*Liu-wei-ti-huang-wan*)	kidney yin *xu* incontinence oliguria dribbling cloudy urine (heat in urine) mouth parched throat dry

URINARY DISORDERS

UPPER HEATER

	Formula	Differentiation
* p. 548	Platycodon & Fritillaria Comb. (*Ching-fei-tang*) plus scute morus	lung heat attacking kidney cough, thirst, chest distress (urine passes in drops) T–thin yellow coat P–slippery, rapid
* p. 196	Rehmannia & Akebia Formula (*Tao-chih-san*)	heat in heart transferring to S.I. reddish urine intermittent, difficult flow mouth dry T–red, cracked insomnia P–rapid
* p. 164	Lotus Seed Combination (*Ching-hsin-lien-tzu-yin*)	if GI weakness and/or watery leukorrhea

MIDDLE HEATER

Chia-wei-wei-ling-tang

peony	1.5 gm	pinellia	1.5 gm	
ginseng	1.5 gm	hoelen	1.5 gm	
agastache	1.5 gm	licorice	3 gm	
crataegus	1.5 gm	polyporus	3 gm	
cyperus	3 gm	fresh ginger	2 gm	
citrus peel	1.5 gm			
atractylodes	1.5 gm			
magnolia	1.5 gm			
alisma	1.5 gm			

damp heat
oliguria w̄ turbidity
full/distressed abdomen
fatigue/heaviness
unwilling to speak
thirst but no desire to drink
P- slippery

	Formula	Differentiation
* p. 260	Ginseng & Atractylodes Formula (*Sheng-ling-pai-chu-san*)	*qi xu* clear to whitish urine difficult to pass
* p. 250	Rehmannia 8 Formula (*Pa-wei-ti-huang-wan*)	diabetic polyuria (w̄ thirst) kidney atrophy cystitis dysuria in the last trimester of pregnancy post-hysterectomy incontinence benign prostatic hypertrophy
* p. 472	Polyporus Combination (*Chu-ling-tang*)	cystitis urethritis severe thirst regular urination

* p. 472	Polyporus Combination (*Chu-ling-tang*) plus	TB in kidney/bladder w̄ hematuria
* p. 433	Tang-kuei 4 Combination (*Szu-wu-tang*)	
* p. 519	Capillaris Combiation (*Yin-chen-hao-tang*)	combined kidney/liver disease w̄ thirst full abdomen oliguria icterus/jaundice
* p. 500	Stephania & Ginseng Comb. (*Mu-fang-chi-tang*)	heart disease/palpitations, dyspnea edema chest distress oliguria
* p. 435	Persica & Rhubarb Combination (*Tao-ho-cheng-chi-tang*)	injury to genitals w̄ oliguria
* p. 472	Polyporus Combination (*Chu-ling-tang*) plus	initial stage gonorrhea
* p. 181	Gentiana Combination (*Lung-tan-hsieh-kan-tang*)	
* p. 291	Minor Cinnamon & Peony Comb. (*Hsiao-chien-chung-tang*)	nocturnal enuresis/nocturia yin *xu* weakness; children
* p. 183	Ginseng & Gypsum Combination (*Pai-hu-chia-jen-sheng-tang*)	high fever/severe thirst polyuria sweating

LOWER HEATER

* p. 472.	Polyporus Combination (*Chu-ling-tang*) or	accumulated heat in bladder painful, dripping urination painful, full abdomen constipation P- slippery, fast, full
* p. 502	Dianthus Formula (*Pa-cheng-san*) or	strong; uro-genital infections acute nephritis
p. 514	Gardenia & Hoelen Formula	urinary stones; urethritis
	single herb: *Polygonum cuspidatum* 15 gm *Hu-zhang-cao*	"accumulated *jing* (sperm) and yin cold" dripping urination fullness lower abdomen = benign prostatic hypertrophy

* p. 250	Rehmannia 8 Formula (*Pa-wei-ti-huang-wan*)	yuan weakness lower heater (*ming men huo*) cold lower abdomen low back pain intermittent urine flow; turbid P- sinking & weak

TONSILLITIS

* p. 395	Pinellia & Magnolia Comb. (*Pan-hsia-hou-pu-tang*) or	difficulty swallowing abnormal sensation in throat 'plum seed *chi*' accumulation of liver *qi* no swelling or pain worse w̄ anxiety: emotional
* p. 160	Bupleurum & Rehmannia Comb. (*Chai-hu-ching-kan-tang*)	if chest distress abdominal tension infantile adenoids
* p. 51	Pueraria Combination (*Ko-ken-tang*) if severe add: platycodon 3 gm gypsum 10 gm	wind-cold attack with sore throat
* p. 347	Licorice & Jujube Comb. (*Kan-mai-ta-tsao-tang*) or	difficulty swallowing; 'plum seed *chi*' with hysteria, GI cramping/upset maybe spasms
	Ginseng & Pinellia Combination (*Qi-qi-tang*) (Seven Chi Soup) pinellia 5 gm ginseng 3 gm cinnamon 3 gm licorice 2 gm fresh ginger 4 gm	if Pinellia & Magnolia ineffective for cold phlegm accumulation anxiety neurosis
p. 603	Platycodon Combination (*Chieh-keng-tang*)	difficulty swallowing due to suppurative swelling sore throat cough w̄ thick phlegm
p. 349	Licorice Combination (*Kan-tsao-tang*)	sore throat but no cough or phlegm

* p. 51	Pueraria Combination (*Ko-ken-tang*) plus Platycodon & Gypsum Comb.	acute tonsillitis
	add pinellia 5 gm	if vomiting
* p. 91	Minor Bupleurum Combination (*Hsiao-chai-hu-tang*) plus Platycodon & Gypsum Comb.	if persists more than 2 days
* p. 91	Minor Bupleurum Combination (*Hsiao-chai-hu-tang*)	chronic tonsillitis
* p. 128	Major Bupleurum Combination (*Ta-chai-hu-tang*) plus Platycodon & Gypsum Comb.	if severe chest distress constipation
* p. 91	Minor Bupleurum Combination (*Hsiao-chai-hu-tang*) plus	if no response & with pain, swelling, infection
* p. 175	Coptis & Scute Combination (*Huang-lien-chieh-tu-tang*) or *Ching-liang-san* (Cleanse and Cool Powder)	esp. viral origin

gardenia	2.5 gm	*tang-kuei*	2 gm
citrus	2.5 gm	fresh ginger	2 gm
kotanon	2.5 gm	platycodon	2 gm
forsythia	2.5 gm	coptis	1 gm
siler	2.5 gm	licorice	1 gm
scute	2 gm	mentha	1 gm

p. 180	Forsythia & Rhubarb Combination (*Liang-ke-san*) plus gypsum 10 gm	chronic tonsillitis with foul breath constipation
* p. 169	Arctium Combination (*Ching-yen-li-ke-tang*)	acute tonsillitis when Pueraria Comb. ineffective and pus remains
p. 619	Platycodon & Chih-shih Comb. (*Pai-nung-san*)	if pus continues to remain

CHRONIC ADENOIDITIS

Page	Formulation	Indications
p. 51	Pueraria Comb. (*Ko-ken-tang*) plus cnidium 2 gm gypsum 5 gm	chronic allergic rhinitis, adenoiditis esp. children prone to ear infections
* p. 91	Minor Bupleurum Combination (*Hsiao-chai-hu-tang*) plus Platycodon & Gypsum Comb.	weaker pt w̄/chest distress white tongue coating
* p. 291	Minor Cinnamon & Peony Combination (*Hsiao-chien-chung-tang*)	if very thin, fatigued nocturia enuresis
	or	
* p. 160	Bupleurum & Rehmannia Comb. (*Chai-hu-ching-kan-tang*)	if chest/abdomen tension
* p. 607	Schizonepeta & Forsythia Comb. (*Ching-chieh-lien-chiao-tang*)	chronic rhinitis/otitis-adults dark, oily skin abdominal tension
* p. 181	Gentiana Combination (*Lung-tan-hsieh-kan-tang*)	if teenager, strong wet fever liver channel
p. 349	Licorice Combination (*Kan-tsao-tang*)	sore throat without suppuration
	or	
p. 603	Platycodon Combination (*Chieh-keng-tang*) platycodon 2 gm licorice 3 gm	if thick phlegm
p. 62	Cinnamon & Mahuang Comb. (*Kuei-chih-ma-huang-ko-pan-tang*) = ½ *Ma-huang-tang* ½ Cinnamon Combination	if w̄ common cold itching no sweating
	Kuei-chih-er-yueh-pi-yi-tang = 2 parts Cinnamon Comb. 1 part Mahuang & Gypsum Comb.	if severe thirst
* p. 72	Mahuang & Asarum Combination (*Ma-huang-fu-tzu-hsi-hsin-tang*)	if common cold in weak pt (combined *shao* yang/*tai* yang conformation) used as preventive in tonsillitis prone
	Decoction of phellodendron bark 5 gm in 300cc boiled to 200cc	preventive antiviral gargle

Page	Formula	Indication
p. 395	Pinellia & Magnolia Comb. (*Pan-hsia-hou-pu-tang*)	sensation of narrowing in throat
p. 351	Cinnamon & Dragon Bone Comb.	if weak, depression palpitations beneath umbilicus
p. 340	Bupleurum & Dragon Bone Comb.	if strong chest distress, shoulder stiff constipation
p. 87	Bupleurum & Peony Formula	if poor appetite afternoon flush shoulder stiff sudden hot/cold sensation
p. 395	Pinellia & Magnolia Comb.	if voice broken, lost weak, cold, tired

Acute Suppurative Tonsillitis

Page	Formula	Indication
p. 169	Arctium Combination (*Ching-yen-li-ke-tang*) "cleanse throat, benefit diaphragm" or *Liu-shen-wan* "Six Spirit Pill" musk, arsenic pearl, borneol crystal bos, licorice bufo	in convulsions esp. children
p. 189	Scute & Cimicifuga Combination (*Pu-chi-hsiao-tu-yin*) or *Chui-hun-hua-tu-tang* "Remove Evil-Transform Toxin Tea" morus, akebia pueraria, bamboo mentha, lonicera licorice, trichosanthes fritillary, achyranthes or	diphtheria dry heat, epidemic redness/swelling/pain throat white membrane spreading throughout throat difficult to remove interferes w̄ breathing

Yang-yin-ching-fei-tang
"Nourish Yin, Cleanse Lung Tea"

rehmannia	30 gm	mentha	7.5 gm
scrophularia	24 gm	moutan	12 gm
ophiopogon	18 gm	peony	12 gm
fritillary	12 gm	licorice	6 gm

VOMITING

****	p. 516	Hoelen 5 Herb Formula (*Wu-ling-san*) vomiting upon drinking water	thirst w̄ vomiting (intestinal flu) gastroenteritis
	p. 483	Alisma, Hoelen, & Ginger Comb. (*Fu-ling-tse-hsieh-tang*)	more severe abdominal symptoms
*	p. 325	Evodia Combination (*Wu-chu-yu-tang*)	migraine w̄ vomiting
	p. 420	*Huang-tu-tang* (yellow oven clay) (Fu-lung-kan Combination)	severe vomiting from rectal obstruction intestinal bleeding
*	p. 110	Pinellia & Ginger Combination (*Sheng-chiang-hsieh-hsin-tang*) "obstruction beneath the heart"	GI gas/foul breath epigastric pain
***	p. 105	Pinellia Combination (*Pan-hsia-hsieh-hsin-tang*)	gastroenteritis food/acute poisoning
*	p. 103	Pinellia & Licorice Comb. (*Kan-tsao-hsieh-hsin-tang*)	severe abdominal cramps
*	p. 395	Pinellia & Magnolia Comb. (*Pan-hsia-hou-pu-tang*)	vomiting from psychological origin; hypersensitive foreign sensation in throat
*	p. 99	Coptis Combination (*Huang-lien-tang*) coptis vs pinellia heat in chest vs pain under heart	vomiting w̄ diarrhea bloody mucus internal heat, chest also gastric hyperacidity; ulcers 1 gm 4 x day
*	p. 295	Ginseng & Ginger Comb. (*Jen-sheng-tang*)	toxic water accumulation stomach spleen yang deficiency excess saliva, diarrhea

	Formula	Indication
* p. 315	Major Zanthoxylum Comb. (*Ta-chien-chung-tang*)	malnourished; low energy vomiting w̄ internal CHILL

DIARRHEA and VOMITING

	Formula	Indication
* p. 516	Hoelen 5 Herb Formula (*Wu-ling-san*)	with thirst
* p. 103	Pinellia & Licorice Comb. (*Kan-tsao-hsieh-hsin-tang*)	with thirst plus severe abdominal cramping
* p. 278	Vitality Combination (*Chen-wu-tang*)	weakness & chronic diarrhea cold limbs
	or	
* p. 313	Aconite & G.L. Comb. (*Szu-ni-tang*)	
	or	
* p. 295	Ginseng & Ginger Comb. (*Jen-sheng-tang*)	

VOMITING with ESOPHAGEAL BLOCKAGE

	Formula	Indication
p. 569	Mume Formula (*Wu-mei-wan*)	due to worms
* p. 555	Pinellia & Gardenia Comb. (*Li-ke-tang*)	due to esophageal cancer mucoid throat obstructions difficulty swallowing
p. 134	Melon Pedicle Formula (*Kua-ti-san*)	due to stagnant food in stomach
* p.. 295	Ginseng & Ginger Comb. (*Jen-sheng-tang*)	due to mucoid esophageal blockage
* p. 295	Ginseng & Ginger Comb. (*Jen-sheng-tang*) =*Li-chung-tang*	stomach chill w̄ no thirst excessive salivation P- slow, sinking
p. 566	Ginseng & Zanthoxylum Comb. (*Li-chung-an-huci-tang*)	stomach chill due to worms ascariasis excess salivation
*** p. 325	Evodia Combination (*Wu-chu-yu-tang*)	stomach-chill w̄ headache

* p. 487	Minor Pinellia & Hoelen Comb. (*Hsiao-pan-hsia-chia-fu-ling-tang*)	stomach-heat, sight of food provokes vomiting pregnancy morning sickness
p. 420	Fu-lung-kan Combination (*Huang-tu-tang*)	severe vomiting w̄ gastric hemorrhage, ulceration
p. 105	Pinellia Combination (*Pan-hsia-hsieh-hsin-tang*) pinellia 5 gm fresh ginger 5 gm	stomach chill w̄ watery sputum water mucus vomit hours after eating chest distress T- white greasy P- slippery
**** p. 212	Magnolia & Ginger Formula (*Ping-wei-san*) add crataegus 1 gm aquilaria 1 gm *shen-chu*	vomiting due to food stagnation foul breath pain after eating (vomiting) persistent bitter taste
* p. 395	Pinellia & Magnolia Comb. (*Pan-hsia-hou-pu-tang*)	vomiting w̄ *qi* accumulation chest distress swollen flanks tired *qi* stuck in throat difficult to swallow
* p. 87	Bupleurum & Peony Formula (*Chia-wei-hsiao-yao-san*) plus aquilaria cardamon saussurea	
* p. 46	Apricot Seed & Perilla Formula (*Hsing-su-san*)	external attack of wind-cold vomiting/dry heaves fever/chill diarrhea
*** p. 100	Agastache Formula (*Huo-hsiang-cheng-chi-san*) children	vomiting w̄ sensation of extreme heat summer colds; gastroenteritis (stagnant food)
p. 569	Mume Formula (*Wu-mei-wan*)	worms in GI; ascariasis vomiting after eating/drinking vomiting bile intermittent abdominal pain esp. w̄ gastric ulceration constant picking of nose huge or no appetite emaciation skin lesions, raised high eosinophyl

Section II
Indications/Differentiation Index by Traditional Chinese Medicine Syndromes

QI DISORDERS

Moving *Qi* Disorders

* p. 493	Atractylodes & Hoelen Comb. (*Ling-kuei-chu-kan-tang*)	flushing up of *qi* headaches/dizziness hysteria/insomnia nervousness/palpitations cinnamon and hoelen main ingredients
* p. 351	Cinnamon & Dragon Bone Comb. (*Kuei-chih-chia-lung-ku-mu-li-tang*)	w̄ umbilical palpitations abdominal spasm/general pain impotence/seminal emission
* p. 340	Bupleurum & Dragon Bone Comb. (*Chai-hu-chia-lung-ku-mu-li-tang*)	chest distress w̄ emotional instability
* p. 85	Bupleurum, Cinnamon, & Ginger Comb. (*Chai-hu kuei-chih-kan-chiang-tang*)	if weaker pt w̄ nervous exhaustion

Combined Moving *Qi* and Stagnant Blood Disorders

* p. 87	Bupleurum & Peony Formula (*Chia-wei-hsiao-yao-san*)	emotional instability/neurosis headaches, flushing up of *qi* menopausal/menstrual irregularity constipation low back discomfort

Stagnant *Qi* Disorders

* p. 395	Pinellia & Magnolia Comb. (*Pan-hsia-hou-pu-tang*)	'Lump stuck in the throat' feeling chest pain/water stagnancy stomach chronic emotional stuckness depression/restlessness
p. 162	Gardenia & Soja Combination (*Chih-tzu-shih-tang*)	chest *qi* stagnation (pain) insomnia, fever irritability in heart below xiphoid
	add licorice 2 gm	if acute palpitations, itching
	add ginger 4 gm	if vomiting

* p. 41	Cyperus & Perilla Formula (*Hsiang-su-san*)	gastrointestinal weakness stomach flu fish food poisoning weakness/food allergies nausea on smell of food
* p. 555	Pinellia & Gardenia Comb. (*Li-ke-tang*)	difficulty swallowing esophageal cancer extreme thirst sticky sputum
* p. 552	Gasping Formula (*Hsiang-sheng-po-ti-wan*)	hoarseness and sore throat nervous laryngitis loss of voice from overuse

In Between Moving *Qi* & Stagnant *Qi*

* p. 386	Gambir Formula (*Kou-teng-san*)	hypertensive w̅ *qi* rising/stiff shoulders hypertensive morning headache abdominal weakness/palpitation obstruction beneath the heart cold limbs/dry skin
* p. 415	Tang-kuei & Gambir Combination (*Chi-wu-chiang-hsia-tang*)	essential hypertension in weak pt w̅ chronic nephritis; arterio-sclerosis flushing up of *qi*/tinnitus heaviness of head
* p. 347	Licorice & Jujube Comb. (*Kan-mai-ta-tsao-tang*)	sedative in hysteria (*qi* rising) insomnia, convulsions, abdominal limbs children's night crying

Qi Formulas to Assist Digestion

Major Four Herb Comb.
Major Six Herb Comb.
Pinellia Combination
Ginseng & Astragalus Comb.

TONIC FORMULAS

	Formula	Indications
* p. 264	Major Four Herb Combination (*Szu-chun-tzu-tang*) = Decoction of 4 Gentlemen add citrus peel to move *qi* through sp/st without accumulation	sp *qi xu*- poor digestion diarrhea/loose stools abdominal distention
* p. 242	Major Six Herb Combination (*Liu-chun-tzu-tang*)	sp yang *xu*- warming action for lethargy, cold limbs
* p. 105	Pinellia Combination (*Pan-hsia-hsieh-hsin-tang*)	accumulated water in stomach w̄ simultaneous vomiting and diarrhea epigastric pain
* p. 295	Ginseng & Ginger Combination (*Jen-sheng-tang*) = *Li-chung-tang* (regulate the middle)	if severe weakness dyspnea spont. sweating indigestion cold limbs

Blood Tonics

	Formula	Indications
* p. 433	Tang-kuei Four Combination (*Szu-wu-tang*)	anemia/general gynecological problems
* p. 585	Tang-kuei & Peony Formula (*Tang-kuei-shao-yao-san*)	any gynecological disorder with weakness/coldness prevention of miscarriage infertility
* p. 576	Tang-kuei & Gelatin Combination (*Chiung-kuei-chiao-ai-tang*)	any chronic uterine (or hemorrhoidal) bleeding
* p. 439	Tang-kuei & Gardenia Combination (*Wen-ching-yin*)	more severe hemorrhagic (heat) manifestations

Qi and Blood Tonics

	Formula	Indications
* p. 248	Ginseng & Tang-kuei 8 Comb. (*Pa-chen-tang*)	general anemia w̄ malabsorption Tang-kuei 4 plus Major Four Herb Comb.
* p. 262	Ginseng & Tang-kuei 10 Comb. (*Shih-chuan-ta-pu-tang*) = "10 Great Supplementing Tea"	more severe weakness post-surgical weakness
* p. 278	Vitality Combination (*Chen-wu-tang*)	severe weakness w̄ water toxicity yin stage cold limbs/diarrhea spont. sweating

poor digestion
general pain/sometimes
paralysis

* p. 239 Ginseng Nutritive Comb.
(*Jen-sheng-yang-yung-tang*)

if chronic exhaustion
w̄ emaciation/palpitations

SHANG HAN LUN FORMULAS

TAI YANG STAGE

Tx: Induce diaphoresis to eliminate surface conformation
herbs acrid, pungent, light
and evaporative in nature
do not overboil
Caution: Excessive induced sweating can cause the collapse of yang.

superficial (*biao*) attack of
exogenous evils
general body ache in the
tendon-muscular meridians
no sweating- strong *wei qi*
fever with chills
neck & shoulder stiffness
first stage of common cold/flu
attacks esp. *tai*-yang channels
(bladder/small intestine)

WIND–COLD Attack

Ma-huang-tang Variations

* p. 76 Mahuang Combination
(*Ma-huang-tang*)

general body ache w̄ headache
fever/chills in strong pt
no sweating
tight chest/difficult breathing
P- floating & full

* p. 66 Mahuang & Coix Combination
(*Ma-hsing-i-kan-tang*)
coix substituted for
cinnamon

muscular rheumatism (myalgia)
predominates; some arthralgia
"water toxin" in surface (muscles)

* p. 68 Mahuang & Apricot Seed Comb.
(*Ma-hsing-kan-shih-tang*)
gypsum substituted for
cinnamon dispels heat

dry asthmatic breathing
predominates (stagnant heat
in lungs w̄ thirst) **but no edema**
flushing up but only mild fever
in strong pt

* p. 81 Major Blue Dragon Combination
(*Ta-ching-lung-tang*)

more severe fever/irritability
restlessness
in strong pt w̄ edema
thirst/headaches/tearing
red eyes

	Formula	Indications
* p. 43	Minor Blue Dragon Combination (*Hsiao-ching-lung-tang*)	less severe fever/flushing up decreased urine milder edema **abdominal fullness** w̄ loose **nausea, dry** stools labored asthmatic cough watery sputum/saliva allergic rhinitis
p. 526	Mahuang and Gypsum Comb. (*Yueh-pi-tang*)	if extreme thirst w̄ **edema** asthmatic cough, oliguria spontaneous sweating predominates
* p. 523	Atractylodes Combination (*Yueh-pi-chia-chu-tang*)	asthma w̄ edema & spont. sweating pain in legs, hands; aversion to chill extreme thirst constipation

Pueraria Combination Variations

	Formula	Indications
* p. 51	Pueraria Combination (*Ko-ken-tang*)	general ache, flushing up type common cold in strong pt stiff neck/spasm predominates no sweating
* p. 50	Pueraria & Magnolia Comb. (*Ko-ken-tang-chia-hsin-i-chuan-chiung*) = Pueraria Comb. + magnolia flower & cnidium	common cold w̄ **nasal congestion** in strong pt w̄ sore throat neuralgia & stiff neck no sweating
	Pueraria Combination plus platycodon 2 gm coix 8 gm	if nasal polyps/congestion with no nasal heat
	Pueraria Combination plus platycodon 2 gm gypsum 10 gm	if nasal polyps/congestion with heat (epistaxis)
* p. 37	Pueraria Nasal Combination (*Ching-pi-tang*)	milder wind-heat w̄ nasal congestion, rhinitis nasal suppuration
	Pueraria Combination plus pinellia 4 gm	common cold-wind-heat w̄ vomiting
	Pueraria Combination plus atractylodes 3 gm aconite ½-1 gm	wind-heat w̄ severe shoulder, neck pain severe chills w̄ cold limbs usually elderly

Non-Mahuang Rhinitis Formulas

* p. 175	Magnolia Flower Formula (*Hsin-i-san*)	nasal congestion, sinusitis
* p. 196	Xanthium Formula (*Tsang-erh-san*)	chronic nasal congestion

Cinnamon Combination Variations

* p. 63	Cinnamon Combination (*Kuei-chih-tang*)	wind-cold/wind-heat in weaker pt spontaneous sweating flushing up of *qi* general body ache, abdominal fullness, **no GI distress**
	add extra cinnamon 6 gm	if severe headache/flushing
p. 58	add pueraria 6 gm Cinnamon & Pueraria Comb. (*Kuei-chih-chia-ko-ken-tang*)	common cold w̄ neck stiffness in weaker pt w̄ sweating
* p. 55	Cinnamon & Astragalus Comb. (*Kuei-chih-chia-huang-chi-tang*)	if excessive sweating; weak constitution tendency to jaundice
p. 54	Cinnamon, Magnolia, & Apricot Seed Combination (*Kuei-chih-chia-hou-pu-hsing-jen-tang*) = Cinnamon Combination plus magnolia bark; apricot seed 4 gm each	if asthmatic cough in pt of weak constitution spontaneous sweating
* p. 351	Cinnamon & Dragon Bone Comb. (*Kuei-chih-chia-lung-ku-mu-li-tang*)	if nervous exhaustion and/or impotence flushing up; vertigo insomnia, palpitations in weak pt w̄ sweating
* p. 302	Cinnamon & Aconite Combination (*Kuei-chih-chia-fu-tzu-tang*)	if cold/chill abdomen dysuria w̄ pain cramping, arthralgia stroke/paralysis pts
* p. 304	Cinnamon & Atractylodes Comb. (with aconite, hoelen) (*Kuei-chih-chia-ling-chu-fu-tang*)	if cold, swollen, painful joints; chronic rheumatism w̄ oliguria sweating

* p. 60	Cinnamon & Peony Combination (*Kuei-chih-chia-shao-yao-tang*)	GI distress/fullness abdominal spasm/diarrhea
p. 124	Cinnamon, Peony, & Rhubarb Comb. (*Kuei-chih-chia-shao-yao-ta-huang-tang*)	if constipation/or diarrhea w̄ tenesmus more severe abdominal distress colitis, dystenery food poisoning
* p. 450	Cinnamon & Anemarrhena Comb. (*Kuei-chih-shao-yao-chih-mu-tang*)	arthritis & rheumatoid pain joint swelling/edema in weak dehydrated pt muscle wasting, atrophy nausea; dry heaves vertigo
* p. 291	Minor Cinnamon & Peony Comb. (*Hsiao-chien-chung-tang*) "Minor support & strengthen the Middle Tea"	yin *xu* heat/fatigue in pt of weak constitution abdominal spasm/pain palpitations tonic for delicate children esp. w̄ flu. gastric ulcers
* p. 76 * p. 63	Mahuang Combination with Cinnamon Combination 50:50	wind-cold chill/body aches with wind-heat sore throat with warm SWEATING in strong pt

SHAO YANG STAGE

* p. 128	Major Bupleurum Combination (*Ta-chai-hu-tang*)	strong pt/muscular or obese severe chest distress constipation shoulder stiffness
* p. 340	Bupleurum, Dragon Bone, & Oyster Shell Combination (*Chai-hu-chia (and)-lung-ku-mu-li-tang*)	mild or no chest distress, nervousness hypertension
* p. 91	Minor Bupleurum Combination (*Hsiao-chai-hu-tang*)	slightly weaker pt alternating fever & chills, white tongue coating
* p. 91	Minor Bupleurum Combination plus Pinellia & Magnolia Combination (*Pan-hsia-hou-pu-tang*)	children's bronchial asthma

	Formula	Differentiation
* p. 117	Bupleurum & Cinnamon Combination (*Chai-hu-kuei-chih-tang*) = Minor Bupleurum Combination plus Cinnamon Combination	weak patient w̄ combined *tai* yang and *shao* yang conformation GI upset chest & abdominal distress - chronic 'cold' in infants - preventive in 'colds' - constipation, abdominal pain - epilepsy in children
* p. 85	Bupleurum, Cinnamon, & (dry) Ginger Combination (*Chai-hu-kuei-chih-kan-chiang-tang*) surface weak - cinnamon inside weak - dry ginger trichosanthes root	weaker patient less chest distress *qi* rising: heavy fullness in head/thirst/palpitation forehead sweat/cold limbs diarrhea or soft stools
* p. 87	Bupleurum & Peony Formula (*Chia-wei-hsiao-yao-san*)	Menopausal disorders fatigue headaches w̄ constipation lumbago emotional instability neurotic cleanliness nagging also: post surgical abdominal pain
* p. 255	Ginseng & Astragalus Combination (*Pu-chung-i-chi-tang*) "Supplement the middle; Strengthen *Ch'i* Tea"	Otsuka Keisetsu: 1st formula to start on any condition where weakness is a major symptom convalescent weakness anemia/anorexia severe prolapse hemorrhoids
* p. 613	Cimicifuga Combination (*I-tzu-tang*)	hemorrhoids prolapse- urogenital itching/pain in genitals
* p. 624	Bupleurum & Schizonepeta Comb. (*Shih-wei-pai-tu-tang*)	urticaria suppurative skin diseases
* p. 609	Schizonepeta & Siler Formula (*Ching-fang-pai-tu-san*)	more severe skin suppuration w̄ chills/fever carbuncles/boils dermatitis
* p. 543	Bupleurum & Scute Comb. (*Chai-hsien-tang*) "Quiet Chest Tea"	very severe chest pain on deep breathing or cough

* p. 35 Bupleurum & Pueraria Comb.
(*Chai-ko-chieh-chi-tang*)
= Minor Bupleurum Combination
plus Pueraria Combination

combined *tai* yang/*shao* yang
conformation
chest distress w̄ shoulder
stiffness
insomnia, headache, fever
dry (or bleeding) nose
thirst & no sweating
chills/painful limbs
use when Mahuang Comb. or
Cinnamon Comb. ineffective

Upper Heater Formulas

Nobose: Flushing/'*qi* rising'
blood congestion in head
red face; irritability
headache/tinnitus
hypertension/arteriosclerosis
dry throat/nasal passages
insomnia
constipation
thirst
"*hsin hsia*" - localized chest distress
under the heart
softness/'turgidity',
slight swelling

actually, upper heater
influencing the
middle heater/stomach

p. 194 Rhubarb Combination
(*Ta-huang-huang-lien-hsieh-hsin-tang*)
'Rhubarb-Coptis Purge the Heart Tea'

mental distress in
firm conformation &
flushing up: mania,
epilepsy, coma

Diff: not used much

* p. 190 Coptis & Rhubarb Combination
(*San-huang-hsieh-hsin-tang*)
'3 Yellow Purge the Heart Tea'
Prevents Stroke

most bleeding conditions
anxiety/fear/flushing
constipation

Diff: **Bupleurum Formulas-**
shoulder pain
hypochondrial chest
distress (costal margin)
flushed face

Coptis & Rhubarb Comb.
no shoulder pain
no chest distress- only
under the heart/local
redder face- more heat

* p. 175 Coptis & Scute Combination
(*Huang-lien-chieh-tu-tang*)

as above if no constipation
all types of bleeding
from excess heat
epistaxis
black tarry stool

		infections of upper heater with great inflammation redness/swelling
* p. 271	Scute Combination (*Tzu-sheng-tung-erh-tang*)	hearing difficulty due to nephrasthenia (ki yin *xu*) tinnitus, elderly drug induced deafness
* p. 439	Tang-kuei & Gardenia Combination (*Wen-ching-yin*) = Coptis & Scute Combination plus Tang-kuei 4 Combination	anemic pt w̄ tendency toward bleeding skin infections w̄ itching much inflammation liver dysfunction stomatitis
* p. 610	Siler & Coix Combination (*Ching-shang-fang-feng-tang-chia-i-yi-jen*) if constipation, must add rhubarb 1 gm or will relapse	acne w̄ facial heat/flushing heat in upper heater also- otitis media gingivitis conjunctivitis red nose
p. 148	Rhubarb & Kan-sui Combination (*Ta-hsien-hsiung-tang*)	damp-heat in chest w̄ pain pulmonary edema/emphysema pulmonary abscess Tx: strong purgation in strong constitution
p. 142	Minor Trichosanthes Combination (*Hsiao-hsien-hsiung-tang*)	concentrated sputum and heat in chest pneumonia/pleurisy intercostal neuralgia gallstones
* p. 543	Bupleurum & Scute Combination (*Chai-hsien-tang*) = Minor Bupleurum Comb. plus Minor Trichosanthes Comb.	sputum & heat accumulated in the heart w̄ heat in the chest palpitations dyspnea chest pain on cough bitter taste T- yellow coat pleurisy/pneumonia hepatitis bronchitis/common cold
* p. 500	Stephania & Ginseng Comb. (*Mu-fang-chi-tang*)	cardiac asthma and edema

p. 480 Hoelen, Apricot, & Licorice (*Fu-ling-hsing-jen-kan-tsao-tang*)
angina pectoris

Middle Heater Formulas

* p. 98 Coptis Combination (*Huang-lien-tang*)
stomach chill clear vomitus
perhaps undigested food
gastroenteritis
bad breath/hyperacidity
abdomen feels cold to touch
cold, clammy sweat
Main use: acute food poisoning
gastric/duodenal ulcer

* p. 105 Pinellia Combination (*Pan-hsia-hsieh-hsin-tang*)
esp. if 'water in stomach'
milder abdominal pain
diarrhea

* p. 103 Pinellia & Licorice Comb. (*Kan-tsao-hsieh-hsin-tang*)
GI distress w̅ emotional instability
hypersensitivity

* p. 110 Pinellia & Ginger Comb. (*Sheng-chiang-hsieh-hsin-tang*)
gastroenteritis w̅ diarrhea
severe water stagnation of st
halitosis

p. 103 Pinellia & Licorice Comb. (*Kan-tsao-hsieh-hsin-tang*)
plus *Prunus mume*
zanthoxylum
stomach chill/water toxin
w̅ excessive saliva

YANG *MING* STAGE

SURFACE-WEAK/INSIDE STRONG Conformation

"Sunlight/Bright Light Stage"
= easily seen stage

Five Approaches to Treatment of Yang *Ming*

disease 'toxin' penetrates
to lower heater- abdomen
'*szu ta zheng*/4 big symptoms'
- big pulse: bounding
- big fever: no chills
- big sweat
- big thirst
- distented abdomen
w̅ constipation
umbilical palpitations

1) Abdominal Fullness
w̅ constipation
Purgation: **Rhubarb Formulas**

2) High Fever w̅ Thirst
'Cleanse Heat':
Gypsum/ Anemarrhena Formulas

3) Heat Remains in the Chest
'Remove Irritability':
Black Fermented Soja Gardenia Formulas

4) Stagnant Blood
Apricot Seed, Moutan,
***Tang-kuei*, Cnidium**
Formulas

5) Irregular Urination: anuria, dysuria, oliguria
'Remove Water':
Hoelen, Alisma, Atractylodes,
Plantago Formulas

FORMULAS

1) Abdominal Fullness with Constipation
Major Rhubarb Combination/*Ta-cheng-chi-tang* p. 145
*Minor Rhubarb Combination/*Hsiao-cheng-chi-tang* p. 141
Rhubarb & Mirabilitum Comb./*Tiao-wei-cheng-chi-tang* p. 154
Rhubarb & Licorice Comb./*Ta-huang-kan-tsao-tang* p. 152
*Apricot Seed & Linum Formula/*Ma-tzu-jen-wan* p. 535

2) High Fever with Thirst
*Ginseng & Gypsum Comb./*Pai-hu-chia-jen-sheng-tang* p. 183
*Sweet Combination/*Kan-lu-yin* p. 177

3) Severe Heat in the Chest
Gardenia & Soja Combination/*Chih-tzu-shih-tang* p. 162
Gardenia, Soja, & Licorice Comb./*Chih-tzu-kan-tsao-shih-tang* p. 161
Gardenia, Soja, & Ginger Comb./*Chih-tzu-sheng-chiang-shih-tang* p. 162

4) Stagnant Blood Plus Heat in the Lower Heater
*Rhubarb & Moutan Combination/*Ta-huang-mu-tan-pi-tang* p. 626
*Persica & Rhubarb Comb./*Tao-ho-cheng-chi-tang* p. 435
*Cinnamon & Hoelen Formula /*Kuei-chih-fu-ling-wan* p. 423
*Tang-kuei & Peony Formula/*Tang-kuei-shao-yao-san* p. 585
*Tang-kuei & Evodia Comb./ *Wen-ching-tang* p. 588
Tang-kuei & Parsley Comb./*An-tai-yin* p. 572
*Tang-kuei & Ginger Comb./*Sheng-hua-tang* p. 583
Rhubarb & Leech Comb./*Ti-tang-tang* p. 437
*Ginseng & Astragalus Comb./ *Pu-chung-i-chi-tang* p. 255
*Lycium Formula/*Huan-shao-tan* p. 237
*Ginseng Nutritive Comb./*Jen-sheng-yang-yung-tang* p. 239

5) Irregular Urination/ Yang *Ming* Water Accumulation
*Hoelen & Alisma Comb./*Fen-hsiao-tang* p. 205
*Hoelen 5 Herb Formula/*Wu-ling-san* p. 516
*Polyporus Comb./*Chu-ling-tang* p. 472
*Hoelen 5 Herb plus Magnolia & Ginger Comb. pp. 516/212
*Hoelen 5 Herb plus Capillaris Comb. pp. 516/519
*Minor Blue Dragon plus Hoelen Comb. pp. 43/486
Atractylodes & Hoelen Comb. p. 493
Tang-kuei & Atractylodes Comb. p. 427

	Ginger & Hoelen Comb.	p. 491
	Hoelen, Licorice, & Jujube Comb.	p. 495
	Hoelen & Locorice Comb.	
	Hoelen, Licorice, & Schizandra Comb.	p. 496
	*Hoelen & Schizandra Comb.	p. 556

Abdominal Fullness with Constipation
Lower Heater Disorders Influencing Entire Body

p. 145	Major Rhubarb Combination (*Ta-cheng-chi-tang*)	stagnancy in all three heaters high fever in strong pt delirium, gasping extreme thirst/nausea tenesmus cold sweating; cold limbs
* p. 141	Minor Rhubarb Combination (*Hsiao-cheng-chi-tang*)	middle heater stagnancy obesity food poisoning/bloating
p. 154	Rhubarb & Mirabilitum Comb. (*Tiao-wei-cheng-chi-tang*)	lower heater stagnancy weaker action than above chronic habitual constipation in men/elderly acute gastroenteritis/food stagnation $\overline{w}$ heat conformation
p. 152	Rhubarb & Licorice Combination (*Ta-huang-kan-tsao-tang*) rhubarb 4 gm licorice 1 gm	simple constipation with **vomiting/gastritis after eating** gastritis vomiting during pregnancy pediatric epilepsy average constitution without fever
* p. 535	Apricot Seed & Linum Formula (*Ma-tzu-jen-wan*) = Minor Rhubarb plus flax seed peony moisturizers apricot seed	chronic heat constipation in weak & elderly pt dry stools
p. 533	Linum & Rhubarb Comb. (*Jun-chang-tang*) 'Moisturize Intestines Tea'	rabbit pellet stools, dry skin

Four Most Commonly Prescribed Constipation Formulas

p. 128	Major Bupleurum Combination (*Ta-chai-hu-tang*)	chest distress hypertension
p. 119	Siler & Platycodon Formula (*Fang-feng-tung-sheng-san*)	obesity general toxicity
p. 190	Coptis & Rhubarb Combination (*San-huang-hsieh-hsin-tang*)	heat in upper heater/flushed hypertension
p. 535	Apricot Seed & Linum Formula (*Ma-tzu-jen-wan*)	elderly, weak w̄ habitual chronic constipation

High Fever with Thirst

* p. 183	Ginseng & Gypsum Combination (*Pai-hu-chia-jen-sheng-tang*)	purge both surface & internal heat due to insufficient moisture must have severe thirst even after drinking reduce fever in flu/cerebritis/pneumonia typhoid/scarlet fever cellulitis sunstroke severe pruritis diabetes w̄ thirst, severe
* p. 177	Sweet Combination (*Kan-lu-yin*)	stomach heat rising to mouth due to heart fire liver yang rising stomatitis/tonsillitis abdominal fullness w̄ internal heat

Severe Heat in the Chest

p. 162	Gardenia & Soja Combination (*Chih-tzu-shih-tang*) Contraindications: DIARRHEA	angina pectoris irritability/insomnia bitter taste/stomatitis mild fever sensation
	add licorice 2 gm	if dyspnea/itching/somatic fever
	add fresh ginger 4 gm	if vomiting

Stagnant Blood and Heat in the Lower Heater

lower heater cold
upper heater hot

- prone to nosebleeds
  - hematuria
  - hemoptysis
- headaches/dizziness
- palpitations/insomnia
- shoulder stiffness
- abdominal fullness

pain in lower left quadrant on abdominal palpation
poor circulation/blood congestion
dark purplish infra-orbital area
dry skin
varicose veins
irregular menses
tinnitus/cold low back
numbness/poor memory/dysuria

	Formula	Indications
* p. 626	Rhubarb & Moutan Comb. (*Ta-huang-mu-tan-pi-tang*)	pain lower RIGHT quadrant in strong pt chronic appendicitis bladder infections/stones gonorrhea/leukorrhea
* p. 435	Persica & Rhubarb Comb. (*Tao-ho-cheng-chi-tang*)	pain lower LEFT quadrant in strong pt blood stagnancy w̄ internal heat severe congestion/heat in head dysmenorrhea/constipation
* p.423	Cinnamon & Hoelen Formula (*Kuei-chih-fu-ling-wan*)	stagnant blood from injuries/ contusions menstrual irregularity in young women, average constitution poor circulation lower body lower back pain upper heater congestion shoulder pain
* p. 585	Tang-kuei & Peony Formula (*Tang-kuei-shao-yao-san*)	weaker anemic pt w̄ heat upper heater less severe abdominal pain
	add ginseng 3-4 gm	if severe weakness
	add coix 10 gm	if poor complexion/dark spots skin 'age spots'
* p. 588	Tang-kuei & Evodia Comb. (*Wen-ching-tang*)	severe cold in reproductive organs cold low back infertility flushing up/dry mouth, lips
p. 572	Tang-kuei & Parsley Comb. (*An-tai-yin*)	strengthen uterus during pregnancy w̄ low back, abdomen pain
* p. 583	Tang-kuei & Ginger Comb. (*Sheng- hua-tang*)	placental retention w̄ postpartum bleeding/stagnant blood

p. 437	Rhubarb & Leech Combination (*Ti-tang-tang*)	old chronic stagnancy; where other formulas ineffective

Water Accumulation Formulas

* p. 205	Hoelen & Alisma Combination (*Fen-hsiao-tang*) most powerful water- removing formula	severe water retention in lower heater (ascites) in strong pt nephrosis severe constipation/gas peritonitis vomiting delayed from drinking water
* p. 516	Hoelen Five Herb Formula (*Wu-ling-san*)	pt must have thirst vomiting just after drinking water stomach flu nephrosis
* p. 472	Polyporus Combination (*Chu-ling-tang*)	dysuria; blood in urine; fever heat in lower heater/severe thirst edema, limbs
p. 516 p. 212	Hoelen Five Herb Formula plus Magnolia & Ginger Comb.	acute gastroenteritis
p. 516 p. 519	Hoelen Five Herb Formula plus Capillaris Combination	combined ki/lv* *xu* w̄ jaundice
p. 91	add Minor Bupleurum Comb.	if more chest distress
* p. 493	Atractylodes & Hoelen Comb. (*Ling-kuei-chu-kan-tang*)	combined *qi* & water disorder vertigo, dizziness; *qi* rising cold feet; oliguria stomach water stagnancy
p. 427	Tang-kuei & Atractylodes Comb. (*Lien-chu-yin*) = Tang-kuei 4 plus Atractylodes Combination	combined *qi xu* & *xue xu* facial edema w̄ anemia, tinnitus vertigo
p. 491	Ginger & Hoelen Combination (*Ling-chiang-chu-kan-tang*)	chill below the waist '*Dai Mo* Conformation' heavy cold legs, as if sitting in water edema of legs, waist freq. urination
p. 495	Hoelen, Licorice, & Jujube Comb. (*Ling-kuei-kan-tsao-tang*)	severe palpitations headaches/dizziness/insomnia vomiting, sweating, more dry heaves flushing up of *qi*

* lv : liver

= cardiac valvular disease
* hysteric palpitation of heart
* labored breathing
* severe abdominal pain
oliguria

p. 496 Hoelen, Licorice, & Schizandra Combination (*Ling-kuei-wei-kan-tang*)

qi rising w̅ palpitations
with **dyspnea**
asthma, cold limbs
emphysema
common cold
*oliguria

flushing up of *qi*/palpitations diff: p. 495

* p. 556 Hoelen & Schizandra Combination (*Ling-kan-chiang-wei-hsin-hsia-jen-tang*)

inside chill w̅ 'water toxin'
in weak, elderly pt
chronic respiratory disease
anemia
palpitations
cold extremities
vomiting
edema, lower limbs

TAI YANG STAGE

serious internal cold
abdomen cold, weak, painful
vomiting
anorexia
diarrhea
P- sinking, slow
small; weak

lower heater syndrome
no fever
extremities warm
abdomen weak & distended
slight pain
vomiting
anorexia
loose stools
no thirst
P- weak, deep
T- white, smooth coat

Tx: Warming & Supplementing

p. 150 Rhubarb & Aconite Comb. (*Ta-huang-fu-tzu-tang*)

coldness in stomach
cold sputum accumulation in chest
unilateral pain,
hypochondrium, waist, legs

p. 124 Cinnamon, Peony, & Rhubarb Comb. (*Kuei-chih-chia-shao-yao-ta-huang-tang*)
= Cinnamon & Peony plus rhubarb

fever w̅ severe chills
abdominal fullness w̅ tenesmus
diarrhea or constipation
colitis
febrile dysentery, food
poisoning; indigestion

* p. 295	Ginseng & Ginger Comb. (*Jen-sheng-tang*)	edema; cold hands/feet excessive salivation/chills chronic but milder symptoms
* p. 291	Minor Cinnamon & Peony Comb. (*Hsiao-chien-chung-tang*)	abdominal pain w̄ spasms extreme *yin xu* heat children w̄ weak constitution

SHAO YIN STAGE

sleeping-exhaustion accumulation of chest HEAT heart irritability early: weak heat-yin *xu* later: cold extremities diarrhea chill; no fever P- slight, small, thin	**Early Weak Fever Conformation** irritable insomnia thirst/sore throat abdominal fullness diarrhea or constipation P- small, rapid T- red **Later Weak Cold Conformation** chills lying fetal position watery diarrhea cold limbs exhausted P- difficult to find T- white coat

* p. 291	Minor Cinnamon & Peony Comb. (*Hsiao-chien-chung-tang*)	yin *xu* heat w̄ abdominal pain w̄ spasm
* p. 72	Mahuang & Asarum Combination (*Ma-huang-fu-tzu-hsi-hsin-tang*)	respiratory distress w̄ internal chills; thin sputum feeble geriatric pt w̄ common cold; influenza pneumonia; bronchitis
* p. 278	Vitality Combination (*Chen-wu-tang*)	exhaustion w̄ GI weakness; internal chills, flushing cold extremities, edema
* p. 313	Aconite, Ginseng, & Licorice Combination (*Szu-ni-tang*)	severe internal chills spontaneous sweating diarrhea; cold limbs edema

Page	Formula	Indications
p. 288	Aconite Combination (*Fu-tzu-tang*)	generalized pain/arthralgia w̄ severe internal chill anemia, sweating, edema diarrhea, numbness

JUE YIN

	Differentiation	Indications
	upper heat; lower cold conformation thirst; irritability T- slightly yellow coat P- rapid, wiry, but thready anorexia or hunger vomits worms	exhausted yin: coldness confused *qi* sensations/flow '*qi* attacks the heart' - irritability; pain cold extremities thirst/dryness
	weak pulse suddenly stronger sudden thirst, hunger w̄ appetite sensation of warmth, alertness	just before death last effort of the yang *qi*
p. 311	Ginger, Licorice, & Aconite Combination with ginseng (*Szu-ni-chia-jen-sheng-tang*)	***Shang han*** diseases, acute vomiting w̄ diarrhea/dysentery cold sweats, extreme weakness cold limbs
p. 321	Tang-kuei & Jujube Comb. (*Tang-kuei-szu-ni-tang*)	if abdominal cramps/spasm
p. 569	Mume Formula (*Wu-mei-wan*)	vomiting of ascariades

YIN STAGE INSIDE-COLD FORMULAS

(LATER SCHOOL)

Page	Formula	Indications
* p. 306	Cinnamon & Ginseng Comb. (*Kuei-chih-jen-sheng-tang*) = Ginseng & Ginger Comb. plus cinnamon	headache w̄ surface heat common cold/flu inside cold; acute gastric enteritis diarrhea/cold feet
* p. 295	Ginseng & Ginger Comb. (*Jen-sheng-tang*)	stomach weak w̄ chills 'water toxicity' vertigo edema/cold limbs/diarrhea

	Formulation	Differentiation
p. 287	Aconite, Ginseng, & Ginger Combination (*Fu-tzu-li-chung-tang*) = Ginseng & Ginger Comb. plus aconite	severe cold severe pain
p. 288	Aconite Combination (*Fu-tzu-tang*)	cold type arthralgia/neuralgia numbness w̄ spont. sweating inside cold; cold limbs general spasm, cramping diarrhea, edema
* p. 278	Vitality Combination (*Chen-wu-tang*) hoelen greater than atractylodes to remove 'water toxin' from stomach	chronic watery diarrhea in weak pt severe fatigue/inside cold stomach 'water toxin' distended w̄ 'splashing' on palpation
* p. 350	Licorice Combination (8 gm) (*Kan-tsao-tang*)	sore throat abdominal pain removes fire; clears toxins warms lungs; dissolves sputum supports the middle; augments *qi* smooth muscle spasm
* p. 108	Peony & Licorice Comb. (*Shao-yao-kan-tsao-tang*)	muscle spasm acute pain
p. 310	Peony, Licorice, & Aconite Comb. (*Shao-yao-kan-tsao-fu-tzu-tang*)	if w̄ severe cold, chill add ½-1 gm aconite to Peony & Licorice (3 gm each)
* p. 298	Licorice & Aconite Combination (*Kan-tsao-fu-tzu-tang*)	severe arthralgia (damp numbness) w̄ swelling, rheumatism dyspnea; fear of chill-wind spontaneous sweating dysuria
p. 300	Licorice & Ginger Combination (*Kan-tsao-kan-chiang-tang*) = *Erh-sheng-tang* "Two-Gods Decoction"	extremely weak/elderly pt w̄ yang *xu*: polyuria enuresis hypersalivation/hiccups weak postpartum/pain
p. 323	Aconite, Ginger, & Licorice Pulse Combination (*Tung-mo-szu-ni-tang*)	absolute yin stage irregular pulse severe cold limbs
p. 311	Aconite, Ginger, & Licorice with Ginseng Comb. (*Szu-ni-chia-jen-sheng-tang*)	exhausted yin stage blood/pus diarrhea cold sweats/fever

p. 283	Hoelen, Ginger, Licorice, & Aconite Combination (*Fu-ling-szu-ni-tang*)	if irritable pt w̄ palpitations & edema ('water toxin on the heart')
* p. 130	Tang-kuei & Magnolia Formula (*Wu-chi-san*) = 'Five Accumulations Powder' blood sputum *qi* cold food	"cold" numbness: chronic rheumatic general body pain upper heater hot-irritable lower heater cold low back pain hernia menstrual pain

CHANG FU SYNDROMES

SPLEEN

p. 264	Major Four Herb Combination (*Szu-chun-tzu-tang*)	gastrointestinal weakness spleen *qi* deficiency
* p. 242	Major Six Herb Combination (*Liu-chun-tzu-tang*)	spleen yang deficiency cold limbs
* p. 255	Ginseng & Astragalus Comb. (*Pu-chung-i-chi-tang*)	spontaneous sweating white frothy mouth/dyspnea rectal prolapse/diarrhea
* p. 260	Ginseng & Atractylodes Formula (*Sheng-ling-pai-chu-san*)	spleen cold damp diarrhea after eating poor circulation fatigue/chills
* p. 516	Hoelen Five Herb Formula (*Wu-ling-san*)	'damp damages the spleen, producing diarrhea'; 'water toxin' in stomach edema/obesity thirst/*qi* rising
* p. 212	Magnolia & Ginger Formula (*Ping-wei-san*) stronger pt; no heat in upper heater/head	stagnant food
p. 234	Saussurea & Cardamon Comb. (*Hsiang-sha-liu-chun-tzu-tang*) = Major Six Herb Comb. plus saussurea 1.5 gm cardamon 1.5 gm	weak pt/elderly 'water toxin' st/sp stagnant food in stomach fullness after eating diarrhea w̄ undigested food Tx: strengthen the spleen; to increase the *qi*

p. 505	Magnolia & Atractylodes Comb. (*Shih-pi-yin*)	**Spleen/Kidney Yang Deficiency** chronic nephritis cardiac edema/fatigue copious, clear urine chills

Damp

* p. 212	Magnolia & Ginger Formula (*Ping-wei-san*)	strong pt w̄ 'water toxin' st w̄ food stagnation nausea
	and/or	
* p. 516	Hoelen Five Herb Formula (*Wu-ling-san*)	if heat in upper heater thirst tendency to obesity/edema

Damp–Cold

* p. 366	Cardamon & Fennel Formula (*An-chung-san*)	weak, anemic pt w̄ st 'water toxin' if severe abdominal pain. gastric ulcer
* p. 91	Minor Bupleurum Combination (*Hsiao-chai-hu-tang*)	if w̄ chest distress
* p. 105	Pinellia Combination (*Pan-hsia-hsieh-hsin-tang*)	if nausea, diarrhea motion sickness, vertigo

Cold

* p. 315	Major Zanthoxylum Combination (*Ta-chien-chung-tang*) more flatulence colon spasm	Tx: warm & supplement the spleen internal chill diarrhea/nausea abdominal pain weak, cold limbs P- weak, slow
	or	
p. 287	Aconite, Ginseng, & Ginger Comb. (*Fu-tzu-li-chung-tang*) *= Ginseng & Ginger Comb. (p. 295) plus aconite ½- 1 gin	less flatulence colon spasm
p. 266	Dioscorea Formula (*Szu-shen-wan*) 'Four Wonders Pill' esp. asthenic children	sp/ki yang *xu* diarrhea before dawn Tx: benefits the *ming men* fire; supplement the earth
	or	

* p. 325	Evodia Combination (*Wu-chu-yu-tang*) psoralea 12 gm schizandra 6 gm myristica 6 gm evodia 4.5 gm fresh ginger 9 gm jujube 6 gm	esp. if chest distress nausea $\overline{w}$ migraine

Heat

* p. 177	Sweet Combination (*Kan-lu-yin*)	sp/st 'hidden fire' always hungry mouth/lips dry, sore throat stomatitis/halitosis irritable constipation possibly dysuria mild jaundice abdominal fullness

STOMACH

Deficiency (*Xu*)

* p. 347	Licorice & Jujube Combination (*Kan-mai-ta-tsao-tang*) or *I-wei-tang* adenophora 9 gm ophiopogon 15 gm *Polygonatum caniculatum* 4.5 gm fresh rehmannia 15 gm sugar crystals 5 gm	**Stomach Yin *Xu*** injured st yin following illness irritable dry mouth anorexia Tx: sweet taste benefits stomach yin hyper-excitability hysteria spastic symptoms
* p. 260	Ginseng & Astragalus Combination (*Pu-chung-i-chi-tang*)	**Stomach Yang *Xu*** indigestion diarrhea after eating anorexia spont. sweating

Tx: increase the yang & benefit the stomach

FOOD RETENTION - Stagnation

Tx: digest food to harmonize the stomach

p. 212	Magnolia & Ginger Formula (*Ping-wei-san*)	fullness after eating halitosis after eating/bitter taste strong pt
p. 110	Pinellia & Ginger Comb. (*Sheng-chiang-hsieh-hsin-tang*)	acid eructation diarrhea neurotic component

Hsiang-sha-chi-chu-wan

chih-shih	3 gm
atractylodes	6 gm
cardamon	3 gm
saussurea	3 gm

FLUID RETENTION - 'Water Toxin'

p. 105	Pinellia Combination (*Pan-hsia-hsieh-hsin-tang*)	epigastric fullness w̄ nausea motion sickness diarrhea
p. 325	Evodia Combination (*Wu-chu-yu-tang*)	if w̄ headaches cold limbs

Cold

p. 315	Major Zanthoxylum Comb. (*Ta-chien-chung-tang*)	abdominal colic w̄ chills heat relieves cold limbs bladder/kidney stones P- slow & weak
p. 325	Evodia Combination (*Wu-chu-yu-tang*)	headache/vertigo vomiting cold limbs
p. 295	Ginseng & Ginger Comb. (*Jen-sheng-tang*)	

Ting-hsiang-shih-ti-san — HICCOUGH when st full; cold stomach; chill

cloves	2.5 gm
persimmon calyx-stem	6 gm (kaki)
ginseng or codonopsis	3 gm
fresh ginger	6 gm

	or Decoction of 20 kaki stems	
* p. 105	**Pinellia Combination**	

Heat

* p. 183	Ginseng & Gypsum Comb. (*Pai-hu-chia-jen-sheng-tang*)	stomach heat always hungry but pt remains thin constant thirst (= diabetes) heaviness/fatigue in limbs
* p. 168	Coptis & Rehmannia Formula (*Ching-wei-san*)	stomatitis/toothache headache
* p. 190	Coptis & Rhubarb Comb. (*San-huang-hsieh-hsin-tang*)	severe heat in head, flushing hematemesis, irritability
p. 145	Major Rhubarb Combination (*Ta-cheng-chi-tang*)	yang *ming* stage/strong pt stomach fullness/pain constipation high fever

LUNG

* p. 537	Ophiopogon Combination (*Mai-men-tung-tang*)	lung yin deficiency high fever red face asthma dry, bleeding throat
* p. 264	Major Four Herb Combination (*Szu-chun-tzu-tang*)	Tx: supplement earth; invigorate metal lu/sp *xu*
	or	
* p. 242	Major Six Herb Combination (*Liu-chun-tzu-tang*)	weak, exhausted anorexia diarrhea
	or	lung deficiency influencing spleen
* p. 493	Atractylodes & Hoelen Comb. (*Ling-kuei-chu-kan-tang*)	
p. 551	Citrus & Pinellia Combination	Tx: nourish the yin **lu/ki yin *xu* of the ki/lu equally** cough w̄ profuse sputum low back pain/discomfort

		seminal emission incontinence P- thready *xu* heat
* p. 253	Lily Combination (*Pai-ho-ku-chin-tang*) or bletilla 3-6 gm/dose	

Damp-Phlegm

p. 595	Lepidium & Jujube Comb. (*Ting-li-ta-tsao-hsieh-fei-tang*) lepidium 1 gm jujube 6 gm	excess sputum/phlegm acute asthma pt cannot lie down

Heat

* p. 173	Morus & Lycium Formula (*Hsieh-pai-san*)	asthma high fever flushed face
* p. 68	Mahuang & Apricot Seed Comb. (*Ma-hsing-kan-shih-tang*)	cough sore throat asthma spontaneous sweating
* p. 576	Tang-kuei & Gelatin Comb. (*Chiung-kuei-chiao-ai-tang*) or indigo 3 gm clam shell 3 gm	cough w̄ hemoptysis painful flanks/chest insomnia
* p. 169	Arctium Combination (*Ching-yen-li-ke-tang*)	cough sore throat/tonsillitis loss of voice
p. 174	Magnolia Flower & Gypsum Comb. (*Hsin-yi-ching-fei-tang*) or Scute & Gardenia Combination (*Huang-chin-ching-fei-yin*) scute 3 gm gardenia 3 flowers	dysuria/anuria accumulated lung heat thirst
* p. 532	Eriobotrya & Ophiopogon Comb. (*Ching-tsao-chiu-fei-tang*)	dry cough w̄ hemoptysis dry, sore throat flushing thirst T– red; no coat P– fast

* p. 395 Pinellia & Magnolia Comb.
(*Pan-hsia-hou-pu-tang*)

weaker pt w̄
GI upset
emotional factors

LARGE INTESTINE

p. 362 Kaolin and Oryza Combination
(*Tao-hua-tang*)

kaolin	6	gm
dry ginger	1.5	gm
oryza	8	gm

large intestine *qi* deficiency
chronic DIARRHEA
weak, cold, elderly
painful abdomen
prolapse/hernia

p. 533 Linum & Rhubarb Combination
(*Jun-chang-tang*)
"Moisten Intestines Tea"

linum	2	gm
tang-kuei	3	gm
chih-shih	2	gm
rhubarb	2	gm
rehmannia, prepared	3	gm
persica	2	gm
scute	2	gm
licorice	1.5	gm
rehmannia, raw	3	gm
apricot seed	2	gm
magnolia bark	2	gm

large intestine dryness
chronic severe CONSTIPATION
'sperm & blood insufficient'
weak, elderly
dry skin

* p. 535 Apricot Seed & Linum Formula
(*Ma-tzu-jen-wan*)
or
Wu-jen-wan
"Five Seed Pill"

pine seed	3	gm
biota seed	9	gm
apricot seed	12	gm
persica (peach seed)	9	gm
Prunus japonicus (seed)	6	gm

plus
citrus peel if stomach heat

chronic severe CONSTIPATION
weak, elderly

Damp-Heat in the Large Intestine

* p. 122 Pueraria, Coptis, & Scute Comb.
(*Ko-ken-huang-lien-huang-chin-tang*)

strong pt, pus & blood in stools

* p. 60	Cinnamon & Peony Comb. (*Kuei-chih-chia-shao-yao-tang*)	weaker pt, abdominal pain

LARGE INTESTINE STASIS - Constipation

* p. 128	Major Bupleurum Combination (*Ta-chai-hu-tang*)	strong pt, chest distress
* p. 535	Apricot Seed & Linum Formula (*Ma-tzu-jen-wan*)	weak pt, dry skin
* p. 405	Perilla Fruit Combination (*Su-tzu-chiang-chi-tang*)	weak pt: normal stool but difficult defecation tense rectus abdominis but full/soft center/navel frequent yawning cold lower limbs
p. 187	Anemone Combination (*Pai-tou-weng-tang*)	damp-heat in large intestine w̄ internal organ toxicity stagnant blood

HEART

* p. 500	Stephania & Ginseng Combination (*Mu-fang-chi-tang*)	**Heart *Qi Xu*** dyspnea palpitations distention beneath the heart edema
* p. 270	Ginseng & Zizyphus Formula (*Tien-wang-pu-hsin-tan*)	**Heart *Yin Xu*** anemia w̄ insomnia palpitations Tx: nourish the heart; pacify the spirit
* p. 351	Cinnamon & Dragon Bone Comb. (*Kuei-chih-chia-lung-ku-mu-li-tang*)	heart and kidney not communicating w̄ nervous exhaustion vertigo seminal emission
* p. 425	Ginseng & Longan Combination (*Kuei-pi-tang*)	**Heart/Spleen Blood Deficiency** Tx: supplement & nourish the he/sp dyspnea insomnia anemia exhaustion

Blood Stagnation

p. 388	Trichosanthes, Bakeri, & Vinegar (*Kua-lou-hsieh-pai-pai-chiu-tang*)	angina pectoris
p. 480	Apricot, Hoelen, & Licorice Comb. (*Fu-ling-hsing-jen-kan-tsao-tang*)	angina w̄/cough, dyspnea

Excess (*Shi*)

Fire

* p. 177	Sweet Combination (*Kan-lu-yin*)	stomatitis, abdominal fullness

Phlegm Misting the Heart – Derangement of the Mind

* p. 395	Pinellia & Magnolia Comb. (*Pan-hsia-hou-pu-tang*)	stuck feeling in throat difficulty swallowing weaker pt
* p. 355	Zizyphus Combination (*Suan-tsao-jen-tang*)	mental exhaustion w̄ insomnia, fatigue weaker pt
p. 114	Bamboo & Hoelen Comb. (*Wen-tan-tang*)	manic phase weak pt neurotic hypersensitivity

SMALL INTESTINE

Deficiency/Cold

* p. 325	Evodia Combination (*Wu-chu-yu-tang*) plus aconite, dry ginger — if severe cold	Tx: warm & smooth the S. I.* severe abdominal pain cold limbs borborgymus
* p. 502	Dianthus Formula (*Pa-cheng-san*)	heart fire transferring to S. I. Tx: cool & purge the S. I. hematuria burning urination constipation

* S. I. : small intestine

LIVER

Deficiency (*Xu*)

Blood Deficiency

	Formula	Differentiation
* p. 432	Tang-kuei Four Combination (*Szu-wu-tang*)	gynecological disorders, anemia
* p. 87	Bupleurum & Peony Formula (*Chia-wei-hsiao-yao-san*)	irritable, anemia flushed, dry skin weak, thirst P–thin, weak
* p. 355	Zizyphus Combination (*Suan-tsao-jen-tang*) or	weak irritable insomnia palpitations night sweats dry mouth/throat
p. 114	Bamboo & Hoelen Comb. (*Wen-tan-tang*) if neurotic hypersensitivity fear/melancholy GI upset	

Liver Yin *Xu*

	Formula	Differentiation
* p. 262	Ginseng & Tang-kuei 10 Comb. (*Shih-chuan-ta-pu-tang*)	Tx: nourish yin & soften the liver irritable insomnia dizziness anger

Stagnation of *Qi* (*Yu*)

	Formula	Differentiation
* p. 91	Minor Bupleurum Combination (*Hsiao-chai-hu-tang*) or	chest distress, tightness thoraco-costal distress stiff neck/thirst/bitter taste palpitations P–wiry T–red w̄ white fur
* p. 395	Pinellia & Magnolia Combination (*Pan-hsia-hou-pu-tang*) or	if emotional component depression weak pt/anemia GI upset "stuck in throat feeling" vertigo

Saussurea & Citrus Formula
(*Mu-hsiang-shun-chi-san*)

saussurea	3	gm
areca seed	3	gm
cyperus	3	gm
citrus peel	3	gm
chih-ko	3	gm
chih-shih	3	gm
cardamon	3	gm
magnolia bark	3	gm
Atractylodes lancea	3	gm (*Cang zhu*)
licorice	1.5	gm

esp. if flanks painful

Stagnation of Blood & *Qi*

I-mu-wan ™ = leonurus 18 gm

abdominal pain
flank pain/meridians-veins painful
general burning sensation

or

* p. 435 Persica & Rhubarb Combination
(*Tao-ho-cheng-chi-tang*)

flushing up of *qi*/dry mouth
shoulder pain
hyper excitable
CONSTIPATION/dysmenorrhea
hypertension/ arteriosclerosis

or

* p. 423 Cinnamon & Hoelen Formula
(*Kuei-chih-fu-ling-wan*)

if NO constipation

Cold in the Liver Channel

* p. 395 Pinellia & Magnolia Comb.

cold on lower heater
GI pain relieved by heat
hernia

or

* p. 409 Lindera Formula
(*Wu-yao-shun-chi-san*)

or

* p. 250 Rehmannia Eight Formula

Liver *Qi* Stagnation with Yang Rising

* p. 128 Major Bupleurum Combination
(*Ta-chai-hu-tang*)

heart, abdomen, flanks painful
strong pt
constipation; yellow tongue fur
GI upset
P- wiry & full
hypertension

	Formula	Indications
		Liver/Spleen *Qi* Stagnation
* p. 87	Bupleurum & Peony Formula (*Chia-wei-hsiao-yao-san*)	Tx: assist the function of Lv/Sp menstrual irregularity flushing of *qi*/insomnia irritable
		Internal Liver Wind
* p. 448	Mahuang & Ginseng Combination (*Hsu-ming-tang*) or	dizziness/irritability swollen eyes/thirst deafness general ache/spasms stroke paralysis facial palsy hypertension
* p. 386	Gambir Formula (*Kou-teng-san*) or	esp. if headaches melancholy dry skin cold hands/feet
* p. 181	Gentiana Combination (*Lung-tan-hsieh-kan-tang*)	if FIRE rising in strong pt urethritis groin lymphadenitis leukorrhea
* p. 183	Ginseng & Gypsum Combination (*Pai-hu-chia-jen-sheng-tang*)	if facial paralysis/neuralgia extreme thirst/dry mouth irritability but fatigue dermatitis abdominal fullness but soft
		Liver *Qi* Harming the Stomach
	Coptis & Evodia Formula (*Tso-chin-wan*) coptis 18 gm evodia 3 gm 9 gm/dose	Tx: purge the liver & harmonize the stomach abdominal pain gastric acid regurgitation

GALLBLADDER

COLD in the Channels

	Formula	Indications
p. 114	Bamboo & Hoelen Combination (*Wen-tan-tang*) weak pt GI upset or	Tx: supplement the gallbladder pacify the spirit fearful easily astonished insomnia palpitations

* p. 355 Zizyphus Combination
(*Suan-tsao-jen-tang*)
weak pt- more fatigue
no GI upset

p. 114 Bamboo & Hoelen Combination
(*Wen-tan-tang*)
plus
cinnamon 2 gm
asarum 2 gm

Tx: warm the gallbladder
move the sputum
concentrated sputum
chest/abdomen discomfort
fear/nightmares
weak heart

DAMP-HEAT

EXCESS (*Shi*)

* p. 519 Capillaris Combination
(*Yin-chen-hao-tang*)

icterus- hepatitis
extreme thirst
chest/abdomen fullness
constipation
dysuria

HEAT

* p. 181 Gentiana Combination
(*Lung-tan-hsieh-kan-tang*)
strong pt only

Tx: cleanse the heat &
purge the gallbladder
eyebrow/temporal headache
pain/fullness lower heater
urogenital heat
symptoms worse after eating
bitter taste/vomiting
anger

* p. 355 Zizyphus Combination
(*Suan-tsao-jen-tang*)
plus deer horn gelatin
bamboo stem
weaker pt

Tx: cleanse the gallbladder
pacify the spirit
heart irritable
insomnia

KIDNEY

Deficiency (*Xu*)

Kidney Yin *Xu*

p. 230 Annemarrhena, Phellodendron, & Rehmannia (6) Formula
(*Chih-po-pa-wei-wan*)
P–weak but big,
deep & superficial

dry tongue/throat
sore throat/thirst
insomnia
anxiety
mild fever

p. 245 Rehmannia 6 Formula
(*Liu-wei-ti-huang-wan*)
P – big & strong

low back pain
incontinence
vertigo/impaired hearing

Kidney *Qi Xu*

p. 359 Lotus Stamen Formula
(*Chin-sou-ku-ching-wan*)

impotence
seminal emission
low back pain
weak legs

p. 351 Cinnamon & Dragon Bone Comb.
(*Kuei-chih-chia-lung-ku-mu-li-tang*)

nervous exhaustion
impotence

Kidney Yang *Xu*

p. 250 Rehmannia Eight Formula
(*Pa-wei-ti-huang-wan*)

cold limbs
seminal incontinence
low back pain/weak limbs

Kidney *Yuan Qi* Weak/Cold

Tx: supplement the marrow & semen

p. 237 Lycium Formula
(*Huan-shao-tan*)

seminal incontinence
impotence
fatigue
anorexia

Kidney Cold - Yang *Xu*

Eucommia & Rehmannia Formula
(*Yu-kuei-wan*)
'Supplement the Right (*Yuan*) Kidney'

rehmannia	8 gm
dioscorea	4 gm
cornus	3 gm
cinnamon	2 gm
aconite	2 gm
tang-kuei	3 gm
lycium fruit	4 gm
deer horn gel	4 gm
eucommia	4 gm
cuscuta	4 gm

Tx: warm & supplement the *yuan qi*

low back cold/discomfort
spermatorrhea
wrist/knees cold, painful
weak legs
stomach pain
diarrhea
frequent urination
impotence
kinetic energy low

p. 288 Aconite Combination
(*Fu-tzu-tang*)
or
Kuei-fu-ti-huang-wan ™

Tx: warm the *ming men*
cold limbs
heaviness in back

p. 278 Vitality Combination
(*Chen-wu-tang*)
if weak gastric/GI
cough
loose stool

Tx: warm & transform *qi*
back pain
cold limbs
irregular urination/edema
fatigue

p. 250 Rehmannia 8 Formula
(*Pa-wei-ti-huang-wan*)
if normal GI-digestion
dyspnea
constipation

Kidney Yin *Xu* (False Heat)

Rehmannia & Achyranthes Formula
(*Tso-kuei-wan*)
'Supplement the Left Kidney'

rehmannia	8 gm
dioscorea	4 gm
cornus	4 gm
lycium fruit	4 gm
deer horn gelatin	4 gm
cuscuta	4 gm
tortoise shell gelatin	4 gm
achyranthes	3 gm

Tx: supplement the yin fluids
tonify the left kidney

dry mouth
thin pale tongue
skin irritation- itching
insomnia
sweating
nocturnal emission
hemoptysis

BLADDER

HEAT

Trigonella & Psoralea Formula
(*An-shen-wan*)™
= 'Peaceful Kidney Pill'

Trigonella foenum	9 gm
Psoralea corylifolia	9 gm
dipsacus	9 gm
melia	9 gm
fennel	9 gm
persica	6 gm
apricot	6 gm
hoelen	6 gm
dioscorea	6 gm

6 gm/dose

heat in the lower heater
dysuria
no thirst
initial urinary tract infection

DAMP–HEAT

	Formula	Differentiation
* p. 472	Polyporus Combination (*Chu-ling-tang*)	cystitis/dysuria/hematuria toxic fever in lower heater extreme thirst/flushing up lower limb edema DIARRHEA
* p. 250	Rehmannia Eight Formula (*Pa-wei-ti-huang-wan*)	nephritis/cystitis back pain cold limbs CONSTIPATION

COLD

	Formula	Differentiation
* p. 516	Hoelen Five Herb Formula (*Wu-ling-san*)	urinary retention slight heat w̄ THIRST vertigo/nausea edema

HEAT and Stagnant Blood

	Formula	Differentiation
* p. 435	Persica & Rhubarb Combination (*Tao-ho-cheng-chi-tang*)	full abdomen/pain low back pain constipation cold feet/burning feeling in upper heater delirium hematuria
p. 437	Rhubarb & Leech Combination (*Ti-tang-tang*)	chronic old blood stagnation lower heater

DAMP–HEAT — Tx: cleanse & moisturize heat

	Formula	Differentiation
* p. 502	Dianthus Formula (*Pa-cheng-san*) or	dysuria hematuria constipation
p. 514	Gardenia & Hoelen Formula (*Wu-lin-san*)	no constipation fever/pain around umbilicus
	Huang-chin-ching-fei-tang coptis 3 gm gardenia 3 flowers or coptis 3 gm scute 3 gm	heat in upper heater with anuria thirst

EIGHT THERAPEUTIC METHODS

I. DIAPHORESIS - Sweating Method

* p. 76	Mahuang Combination (*Ma-huang-tang*)	wind-cold/warm and pungent herbs
p. 58	Cinnamon & Pueraria Comb. = Minor Pueraria Combination (*Kuei-chih-chia-ko-ken-tang*)	
* p. 78	Morus & Chrysanthemum Comb. (*Sang-chu-yin*) or	wind-heat/pungent-cool herbs mild fever, thirst
p. 68	Mahuang & Apricot Seed Comb. (*Ma-hsing-kan-shih-tang*)	
* p. 72	Mahuang & Asarum Combination (*Ma-huang-fu-tzu-hsi-hsin-tang*)	wind cold in yang *xu* pt/cold limbs, profuse phlegm
* p. 81	Major Blue Dragon Combination (*Ta-ching-lung-tang*)	remove water (edema) & induce sweating- strong pt more severe wind-cold: water secretions
* p. 126	Ginseng & Perilla Combination (*Sheng-su-yin*)	nourish blood & induce sweating anemia - weaker pt gastric upset/weak cough
* p. 41	Cyperus & Perilla Formula (*Hsiang-su-san*)	regulate *qi*, disperse st stagnation, & induce sweating GI weakness w̄ common cold
* p. 119	Siler & Platycodon Formula (*Fang-feng-tung-sheng-san*)	dissolve the surface & purge the inside common cold w̄ habitual constipation/auto-intoxication

II. EMESIS

p. 134	Melon Pedicle Formula (*Kua-ti-san*) melon pedicle (stem) 1 gm phaseolus seed 1 gm black fermented soja 5 gm	coldness w̄ heat toxin in upper heater

	if ineffective: small amount of musk by mouth	
p. 135	Ginseng Rhizome Combination (*Sheng-lu-yin*) ginseng rootlets 3-6 gm	slow vomiting in weak pt strong toxin
p. 336	Gleditsia & Asarum Formula (*Tung-kuan-san*) gleditsia 3 gm asarum 3 gm place on upper lip under nostrils	sneezing & expectoration resuscitation of unconscious pt (stroke)

III. PURGATION

	Cheng Chi Formulas	**Attacking the Lower Heater**
* p. 141	Minor Rhubarb Comb. (*Hsiao-cheng-chi-tang*)	constipation/abdominal fullness tidal fever sweating, strong pt
p. 145	Major Rhubarb Comb. (*Ta-cheng-chi-tang*)	more severe high fever delirium
p. 154	Rhubarb & Mirabilitum Comb. (*Tiao-wei-cheng-chi-tang*)	weaker pt/asthma food stagnation; enteritis
* p. 435	Persica & Rhubarb Comb. (*Tao-ho-cheng-chi-tang*)	w̄ blood stagnation; cramping menstrual irregularity cold feet
p. 150	Rhubarb & Aconite Comb. (*Ta-huang-fu-tzu-tang*)	abdominal pain, cold limbs
* p. 535	Apricot Seed & Cannabis Formula Apricot Seed & Linum Formula (*Ma-tzu-jen-wan*)	Tx: increase moisture in lower heater to lubricate habitual constipation in weak/elderly pt
	Aquilaria & Rhubarb Formula (*Kun-tan-wan*) chlorite 12 gm scute 9 gm aquilaria 4.5 gm rhubarb 9 gm 3-6 gm/dose	Tx: attack SPUTUM tenacious, deep sputum

IV. HARMONIZING

Regulate *Hsiao* Yang Exogenous Invasion

* p. 91	Minor Bupleurum Combination (*Hsiao-chai-hu-tang*)	chest distress w̄ nausea bitter taste alternate chills/fever
* p. 128	Major Bupleurum Combination (*Ta-chai-hu-tang*)	more severe chest distress constipation
* p. 85	Bupleurum, Cinnamon, & (Dry) Ginger Combination (*Chai-hu-kuei-chih-kan-chiang-tang*)	weaker pt loose stools
* p. 117	Bupleurum & Cinnamon Comb. (*Chai-hu-kuei-chih-tang*)	weak pt; mild distress w̄ arthralgia

Harmonize Stomach and Spleen

* p. 112	Bupleurum & Chih-shih Formula (*Szu-ni-san*)	chest distress w̄ GI spasm mild chilling limbs neurotic hypersensitivity

V. WARMING

Tx: remove cold evil & supplement yang
diarrhea, edema, cold limbs

* p. 278	Vitality Combination (*Chen-wu-tang*)	Tx: remove cold evil & supplement yang diarrhea, edema, cold limbs
* p. 319	Tang-kuei, Evodia, & Ginger Comb. (*Tang-kuei-szu-ni-chia-wu-chu-yu-sheng-chiang-tang*)	more severe chill cyanotic extremities
* p. 295	Ginseng & Ginger Combination (*Jen-sheng-tang*)	very weak w̄ loose stools gastric fullness
* p. 325	Evodia Combination (*Wu-chu-yu-tang*)	stomach chill w̄ headache vertigo nausea
* p. 315	Major Zanthoxylum Combination (*Ta-chien-chung-tang*)	abdominal chill/nausea colon spasticity
* p. 60	Cinnamon & Peony Combination (*Kuei-chih-chia-shao-yao-tang*)	in weak constitution diarrhea/spastic abdominal colon pain sweating

VI. CLEARING/DISPERSING

Formula	Differentiation
p. 170 Rhinoceros & Rehmannia Comb. (*Hsi-chiao-ti-huang-tang*) substitute 10 gm water buffalo horn for 1 gm rhino horn	salty-cold drugs cleanse blood high fever w/impaired consciousness hemorrhage
* p. 177 Sweet Combination (*Kan-lu-yin*)	nourish the yin & cleanse heat general fever stomatitis sore throat/halitosis
p. 330 Bos & Curcuma Formula (*An-kung-niu-huang-wan*)™	cleanse fever & open orifices of the head fever-toxin type COMA encephalitis, septicemia infectious hepatitis cerebral injury coma summer heatstroke
* p. 386 Gambir Formula (*Kou-teng-san*)	cleanse heat & stop convulsions arteriosclerosis/hypertension epilepsy/CVA
* p. 183 Ginseng & Gypsum Combination (*Pai-hu-chia-jen-sheng-tang*)	hot & cold drugs together cleanse the *qi* high fever of unknown origin
* p. 175 Coptis & Scute Combination (*Huang-lien-chieh-tu-tang*) or * p. 190 Coptis & Rhubarb Combination (*San-huang-hsieh-hsin-tang*)	bitter & cold drugs together cleanse the fire flushing; hemorrhage intracardiac fullness
Rhinoceros & Scrophularia Comb. (*Ching-ying-tang*) rhino horn, coptis rehmannia (fresh), salvia scrophularia, ophiopogon bamboo leaf, forsythia lonicera all 4-6 gm	cleanse blood of internal heat fast pulse reddish-brown dry tongue skin rashes high fever delirium

VII. SUPPLEMENTING (Tonics)

	Formula	Indications
* p. 264	Major Four Herb Combination (*Szu-chun-tzu-tang*) sp/st *xu*	supplement *qi*; weak digestion
* p. 255	Ginseng & Astragalus Combination (*Pu-chung-i-chi-tang*) sp/st/lu *xu*; sputum frothy; spont. sweating	spontaneous sweating; exhaustion; organ prolapse
* p. 433	Tang-kuei Four Combination (*Szu-wu-tang*)	supplement blood
* p. 239	Ginseng Nutritive Combination (*Jen-sheng-yang-yung-tang*)	emaciation, sweating
* p. 270	Ginseng & Zizyphus Formula (*Tien-wang-pu-hsin-tan*) sp/st/he yin *xu*; emotional instability; amnesia	supplement yin
*p. 250	Rehmannia Eight Formula (*Pa-wei-ti-huang-wan*)	supplement yang; cold limbs; low back pain

VIII. REDUCING or DISPERSING

	Formula	Indications
* p. 212	Magnolia & Ginger Formula (*Ping-wei-san*)	food accumulation in strong pt; poor digestion, loose stools
* p. 548	Platycodon & Fritillary Comb. (*Ching-fei-tang*)	remove phlegm & transform water; thick sputum; dry, sore throat
* p. 205	Hoelen & Alisma Combination (*Fen-hsiao-tang*) = Magnolia & Ginger Comb. plus Hoelen & Polyporus Comb.	remove water & disperse swelling; ascites in strong pt

Appendix I
Formula Listings by Therapeutic Methods

1
Chieh Piao Chi
(解表劑 , Sudorific Formulas)

Formulas that promote sweating, relieve muscular tension, speed the eruption of measles, and eliminate surface conformations are called *chieh piao chi*. Such formulas are of the "sweating" method, one of eight major therapeutic methods in Chinese medicine.

A sudorific formula expels toxins accumulated on the surface of the body (skin and hair) that have not yet penetrated to the interior. Expulsion of toxins occurs by means of sweating. The *Shang han lun* says, "He who is proficient at treatment always treats the skin and hair." Any injury, caused by the six excesses generally manifests itself on the surface; hence it is a surface conformation. At this stage, the injurious toxin still light and shallow, can be eliminated by sudorifics which induce sweating, thus dispelling the toxins. The sweating method often precedes other therapeutic methods.

Because most sudorific formulas contain herbs that are acrid, dispersant, light, and evaporative, they should not be overcooked because it causes reduction in effectiveness. At the same time patients treated with a sudorific formula should avoid drafts and the cold and put on more clothes to induce more sweating. Strong sudorifics cause the patient to become soaked with sweat. Note: If there is too little sweating, the toxin is not totally expelled. But excessive sweating may injure normal *ch'i* causing yang to collapse.

Chieh Piao Chi
Qie Biao Qi Sudorific Formulas
Expulsion of surface 'toxins' by sweating

* Bupleurum & Pueraria Combination	*Chai-Ko-Chieh-Chi-Tang* *Chai-Go-Qie-Qi-Tang*
* Pueraria Nasal Combination	*Ching-Pi-Tang* *Zhing-Bi-Tang*

Chiang-huo Combination	*Chiu-Wei-Chiang-Huo-Tang* *Jiu-Wei-Jiang-Huo-Tang*
* Cnidium & Tea Formula	*Chuan-Chiung-Cha-Tiao-San* *Juan-Jiong-Cha-Tao-San*
* Cyperus & Perilla Formula	*Hsiang-Su-San* *Xiong-Su-San*
* Minor Blue Dragon Comb.	*Hsiao-Ching-Lung-Tang* *Shao-Qing-Long-Tang*
* Apricot Seed & Perilla Formula	*Hsing-Su-San* *Xing-Su-San*
* Mahuang & Morus Formula	*Hua-Kai-San* *Hua-Gai-San*
* Ginseng & Mentha Formula	*Jen-Sheng-Pai-Tu-San* *Ren-Shen-Bai-Tu-San*
* Pueraria & Magnolia Comb.	*Ko-Ken-Chia-Hsin-I-Chuan-Chiung* *Ge-Gen-Jia-Xin-I-Quan-Qiong*
* Pueraria Combination	*Ko-Ken-Tang* *Ge-Gen-Tang*
Cinnamon, Magnolia, & Apricot Seed Combination	*Kuei-Chih-Chia-Hou-Pu-Hsing-Jen-Tang* *Gui-Qie-Jia-Hou-Po-Xing-Ren-Tang*
* Cinnamon & Astragalus Comb.	*Kuei-Chih-Chia-Huang-Chi-Tang* *Gui-Qie-Jia-Huang-Qi-Tang*
Cinnamon & Pueraria Comb.	*Hsiao-Ko-Ken-Tang/Kuei-Chih-Chia-Ko-Ken-Tang* *Shao-Ge-Gen-Tang/Gui-Qie-Jia-Ge-Gen-Tang*
* Cinnamon & Peony Comb.	*Kuei-Chih-Chia-Shao-Yao-Tang* *Gui-Qie-Jia-Shao-Yao-Tang*
Cinnamon & Mahuang Comb.	*Kuei-Chih-Ma-Huang-Ko-Pan-Tang* *Gui-Qie-Ma-Huang-Ge-Pan-Tang*
* Cinnamon Combination	*Kuei-Chih-Tang* *Gui-Qie-Tang*
* Mahuang & Coix Combination	*Ma-Hsing-I-Kan-Tang* *Ma-Xing-I-Gan-Tang*
Mahuang & Apricot Seed Comb.	*Ma-Hsing-Kan-Shih-Tang* *Ma-Xing-Gen-Shi-Tang*
Mahuang & Atractylodes Comb.	*Ma-Huang-Chia-Chu-Tang* *Ma-Huang-Jia-Zhu-Tang*

* Mahuang & Asarum Combination	*Ma-Huang-Fu-Tzu-Hsi-Hsin-Tang* *Ma-Huang-Fu-Zi-Xi-Xin-Tang*
Mahuang, Aconite, & Licorice Comb.	*Ma-Huang-Fu-Tzu-Kan-Tsao-Tang* *Ma-Huang-Fu-Zi-Gan-Cao-Tang*
* Mahuang Combination	*Ma-Huang-Tang* *Ma-Huang-Tang*
* Morus & Chrysanthemum Comb.	*Sang-Chu-Yin* *Sang-Zhu-Yin*
* Mahuang & Cimicifuga Comb.	*Shih-Shen-Tang* *Shi-Shen-Tang*
* Major Blue Dragon Combination	*Ta-Ching-Lung-Tang* *Da-Qing-Long-Tang*
* Lonicera & Forsythia Formula	*Yin-Chiao-San* *Yin-Qiao-San*

2
Ho Chieh Chi
(和解劑 , Harmonizing Formulas)

Formulas that eliminate toxins by coordinating the liver and spleen or the stomach and intestines are said to "harmonize." The "harmonizing" method is one of the eight major Chinese healing methods. This type of formula is contraindicated when the harmful toxin remains on the surface and the condition has not entered the lesser yang stage, or when the toxin has entered the interior but sunlight yang fever is thriving. Also, harmonizing formulas are not advisable for persons who are fatigued, have internal injuries, irregular diets, weakness in *ch'i* and blood, or fever and chills.

Ho Chieh Chi
He Qie Qi Harmonizing Formulas—detoxify by coordinating wood with earth (liver with spleen)

* Agastache Formula	*Huo-Hsiang-Cheng-Chi-San* *Ho-Xiang-Cheng-Qi-San*
* Bupleurum & Chih-shih Formula	*Szu-Ni-San* *Si-Ni-San*
* Bupleurum, Cinnamon, & Ginger Combination	*Chai-Hu-Kuei-Chih-Kan-Chiang-Tang* *Chai-Hu-Gui-Zhi-Gan-Zhiong-Tang*
* Bupleurum & Peony Formula	*Chia-Wei-Hsiao-Yao-San* *Chia-Wei-Shao-Yao-San*
* Bupleurum & Tang-kuei Formula	*Hsiao-Yao-San* *Shao-Yao-San*
* Cardamon Combination	*Liu-Ho-Tang* *Liu-Ho-Tang*
* Coptis Combination	*Huang-Lien-Tang* *Huang-Lian-Tang*

* Coptis & Gelatin Combination	*Huang-Lien-Ah-Chiao-Tang* *Huang-Lian-E-Jiao-Tang*
* Minor Bupleurum Combination	*Hsiao-Chai-Hu-Tang* *Shao-Chai-Hu-Tang*
* Pinellia Combination	*Pan-Hsia-Hsieh-Hsin-Tang* *Ban-Xia-Xie-Xin-Tang*
* Pinellia & Ginger Combination	*Sheng-Chiang-Hsieh-Hsin-Tang* *Sheng-Jiang-Xie-Xin-Tang*
* Pinellia & Licorice Comb.	*Kan-Tsao-Hsieh-Hsin-Tang* *Gan-Cao-Xie-Xin-Tang*
Bamboo & Ginseng Combination	*Chu-Ju-Wen-Tan-Tang* *Zhu-Ru-Wen-Dan-Tang*
Scute & Licorice Combination	*Huang-Chin-Tang* *Huang-Qin-Tang*
Bamboo & Hoelen Combination	*Wen-Tan-Tang* *Wen-Dan-Tang*

3
Piao Li Shuang Chieh Chi
(表裏雙解劑 , Dual Dissolving Formulas)

Formulas that treat both the surface and the interior at the same time or have a dissolving action in the interior as well as on the exterior are called *piao li shuang chieh chi.*

The basic rules of treatment are to induce sweating for surface diseases and use purgatives or fever-reducing herbs for interior diseases. If the illness is both external and internal, the surface must be treated first and the interior second. However, if the surface condition has not been fully cured but the interior needs immediate treatment, then a dual surface-interior formula is suggested so that the injurious toxin can be dispelled at once. Formulas are prescribed according to whether the conformation is chill or fever, weak or firm. Formulas of this type are classified as a surface-dissolving, interior-attacking; surface-dissolving, interior-cleansing; or surface-dissolving, interior-warming. However, dual formulas are not for all surface-interior diseases. The treatment of disease and selection of a formula depend on the severity of the person's condition and on the priority of treatment. After the severity and priority of the surface and the interior have been determined, dosage proportions between the surface and the internal drugs are then calculated to avoid excessive or inadequate dosing.

Piao Li Shuang Chieh Chi
Biao Li Shuang Qie Qi Surface and Interior Coordinating Formulas

* Bupleurum & Cinnamon Combination	*Chai-Hu-Kuei-Chih-Tang* *Chai-Hu-Gui-Zhi-Tang*
* Ginseng & Perilla Combination	*Sheng-Su-Yin* *Sheng-Su-Yin*
* Major Bupleurum Combination	*Ta-Chai-Hu-Tang* *Da-Chai-Hu-Tang*
* Pueraria, Coptis, & Scute Combination	*Ko-Ken-Huang-Lien-Huang-Chin-Tang* *Ge-Gen-Huang-Lian-Huang-Jin-Tang*

* Siler & Platycodon Combination	*Fang-Feng-Tung-Sheng-San* *Fang-Feng-Tong-Sheng-San*
* Tang-kuei & Magnolia Combination	*Wu-Chi-San* *Wu-Jia-San*
Magnolia Seven Combination	*Hou-Pu-Chi-Wu-Tang* *Hou-Po-Qi-Wu-Tang*
Cinnamon, Peony, & Rhubarb Combination	*Kuei-Chih-Chia-Shao-Yao-Ta-Huang-Tang* *Gui-Zhi-Jia-Shao-Yao-Da-Huang-Tang*
Gypsum, Coptis, & Scute Combination	*San-Huang-Shih-Kao-Tang* *San-Huang-Shi-Gao-Tang*

4.
Yung Tu Chi
(涌吐劑 , Emetics)

Any formula capable of inducing vomiting is a *yung tu chi* remedy. An emetic causes the patient to vomit sputum, undigested foods, and toxins lodged in the throat, chest, or stomach. The main indications are apoplexy, congestion, fainting, indigestion, poisonous foods, throat paralysis, acute jaundice, dry cholera, and accidental ingestion of poison.

When taking an emetic, the patient must avoid drafty rooms, because vomiting often leaves the patient physically weak and vulnerable to catching cold. If vomiting does not occur after taking the emetic, stimulation of the throat with the hand or a goose feather, or drinking large amounts of water may help.

Should continuous vomiting occur after taking the emetic, ginger juice, cold congee, or cold water will usually arrest the vomiting. However, if vomiting still continues, countermeasures are necessary. For example, 30mg-60mg of musk is an antidote for incessant vomiting resulting from taking *Kua-ti-san* (瓜蒂散 Melon Pedicle Formula). A thick decoction of scullion white treats vomiting induced by *San-sheng-san* (三聖散 Siler and Veratrum Formula). A licorice and aspis decoction arrests vomiting caused by *Hsi-yen-san* (稀涎散 Gleditsia and Alum Formula).

After the vomiting has ceased, stomach upset can be soothed by taking congee to correct inverted *ch'i.* Oily, fried foods or indigestable foodstuffs should be avoided, otherwise the condition may be exacerbated, further injuring the normal *ch'i.*

Although the emetic formula has prompt curative effects for urgent conformations, it can have various harmful effects on the stomach. Therefore, this method of treatment should never be used on weak, debilitated, or elderly patients; it is also prohibited for patients with agitated *ch'i* in the abdomen and inadequacy of *ch'i* and blood; for pregnant women; for persons with amnesia; for patients with hemoptysis (hemorrhage of the larynx, trachea, bronchi or lungs); or for patients with cardiac disease or hypertension.

Yung Tu Chi
 Yung Tu Qi Emetic Formulas

Melon Pedicle Formula	*Kua-Ti-San* *Gua-Di-San*
Siler & Veratrum Combination	*San-Sheng-San* *San-Sheng-San*
Ginseng Rhizome Combination	*Sheng-Lu-Yin* *Sheng-Lu-Yin*
Croton & Apricot Seed Combination	*Tsou-Ma-Tang* *Zou-Ma-Tang*

5
Kung Li Chi
(攻裏劑, Interior Attacking Formulas)

Formulas that attack firmness in the interior of the body are called *kung li chi* or *hsieh hsia chi* (瀉下劑) or purgatives. Purgation is another of the eight major Chinese therapeutic methods.

Purgatives lubricate the intestines, promote bowel movements, eliminate congestion and stagnancy within the stomach and intestines, and decrease edematous swelling of the abdomen or chest.

Purgatives are used for treating firm fever, congestion in the stomach and intestines, dry stools, constipation, stagnated water (fluid) inside the body, or chill accumulation. All of these symptoms are caused by "evil firmness." They can be treated with an interior attacking formula if the patient still has normal vitality.

In prescribing an emetic formula the following precautions need be observed. First, if surface toxin has not been dispelled and the interior is not firm enough, treatment must be carried out according to the rule of surface-first, interior-second. Only after surface toxin has been eliminated and the interior has become firm can a purgative be prescribed. If the surface is not yet cured but the interior has become firm, then, depending on the relative severity of the two, a properly adjusted dual surface-interior attacking formula must be used.

Second, in prescribing purgatives, not only the firmness conformation must be considered but also the weakness conformation. Generally if the patient has a strong tendency toward interior firmness (sound functioning of internal organs), purgation is instituted. If the patient is more inclined to the weakness, then both purgating and supplementing methods are used. Sometimes when constipation is a symptom of the conformation, it should not be treated with a purgative. This prohibition applies especially to physically weak geriatric patients, postpartal women with blood weakness (anemia), recovering patients with inhibited salivation and patients who have lost considerable blood. This type of formula is contraindicated for pregnant women.

Third, most purgatives are injurious and exhaust normal stomach *ch'i* (vitality). Hence their administration should be suspended once they have taken effect, and the patient given a nourishing formula. The patient must be cautioned against eating oily and indigestible foods.

Kung Li Chi
Gung Li Qi Purgative Formula

Platycodon & Croton Formula	*Chieh-Keng-Pai-San* *Qie-Geng-Bai-San*
* Minor Rhubarb Combination	*Hsiao-Cheng-Chi-Tang* *Shao-Cheng-Qi-Tang*
Minor Trichosanthes Combination	*Hsiao-Hsien-Hsiung-Tang* *Shao-Xien-Xiong-Tang*
Rhubarb, Ginger, & Croton Formula	*San-Wu-Pei-Chi-Wan* *San-Wu-Pei-Qi-Wan*
Jujube Combination	*Shih-Tsao-Tang* *Shi-Cao-Tang*
Major Rhubarb Combination	*Ta-Cheng-Chi-Tang* *Da-Cheng-Qi-Tang*
Rhubarb & Kan-sui Combination	*Ta-Hsien-Hsiung-Tang* *Da-Xien-Xiong-Tang*
Rhubarb & Aconite Combination	*Ta-Huang-Fu-Tzu-Tang* *Da-Huang-Fu-Zi-Tang*
Rhubarb & Licorice Combination	*Ta-Huang-Kan-Tsao-Tang* *Da-Huang-Gan-Cao-Tang*
Rhubarb & Mirabilitum Combination	*Tiao-Wei-Cheng-Chi-Tang* *Tiao-Wei-Cheng-Qi-Tang*
Croton & Hematite Formula	*Tzu-Yuan* *Zi-Yuan*

6
Ching Je Hsieh Huo Chi
(清熱瀉火劑 , Fever Cleansing and Fire Purging Formulas)

Formulas composed of chilly and cool herbs treat fever or fire conformations and are called *ching je hsieh huo chi.* This "cleansing" method is another of eight Chinese therapeutic methods. This type of formula is used when a harmful toxin results in a fever. If the injurious fever toxin is on the body surface, it should be treated by sweating; if the fever is internal and the patient firm, purgatives should be used. These formulas are used only after sweating but before the fever has subsided, or when the internal fever is flourishing and is not firm. Only under these conditions can the formula subjugate the fever and result in healing.

A fire-fever conformation is typed according to domain: blood, *ch'i,* firmness and weakness, or organs affected. Therefore, treatment methods also are classified according to those that reduce fever in the *ch'i* domain, those that reduce fever in the blood vessels and blood, those that clean both the *ch'i* and blood, those that purge fire and poisons, and those that reduce visceral and weakness fever.

In prescribing this type of formula certain precautions must be taken. It must be clearly determined whether the fever is genuine or false. A high-grade, short-term fever that expels toxins is termed a real fever whereas a low-grade, persistent fever–such as found in tuberculosis–is deemed a false fever. The same applies to chills. For example, a real-fever, false-chills condition should be treated with a fever-cleansing, fire-purging formula, not with a warming formula, and a false-fever, real-chills condition must be treated with an interior-warming, yang-restoring formula and not with a chill and cool formula.

The dosage must be adjusted to comply with the patient's condition and physical strength. Fever toxin (infection) is liable to reduce or diminish bodily fluids including saliva. Likewise, chilly and cool formulas may cause the harmful toxin to linger and are also deleterious to the stomach and spleen.

If repetitive treatment with fever-cleansing, fire-purging formulas does not bring about a remission of the fever, the condition is considered a conformation which Wang Ping described thusly: "If all efforts fail to lower the fever, it is due to a lack of water (dehydration)." The correct way of treating this kind of conformation is to nourish the yin and augment the water. As the yin is restored, the fever will decrease spontaneously.

Ching Je Hsieh Huo Chi
Qing Re Xue Huo Qi Formulas for "clearing heat" (Fever) by cold herbs

* Arctium Combination	*Ching-Yen-Li-Ke-Tang* *Qing-Yen-Li-Ge-Tang*
* Bupleurum & Rehmannia Combination	*Chai-Hu-Ching-Kan-Tang* *Chai-Hu-Jing-Gan-Tang*
* Cinnamon 5 Herb Combination	*Kuei-Chih-Wu-Wu-Tang* *Gui-Qie-Wu-Wu-Tang*
* Coptis & Rehmannia Formula	*Ching-Wei-San* *Qing-Wei-San*
* Coptis & Rhubarb Combination	*San-Huang-Hsieh-Hsin-Tang* *San-Huang-Xie-Xin-Tang*
* Coptis & Scute Combination	*Huang-Lien-Chieh-Tu-Tang* *Huang-Lian-Qie-Tu-Tang*
Gardenia, Ginger, & Soja Combination	*Chih-Tzu-Sheng-Chiang-Shih-Tang* *Zhi-Zi-Sheng-Jiang-Shi-Tang*
Gardenia, Licorice, & Soja Combination	*Chih-Tzu-Kan-Tsao-Shih-Tang* *Zhi-Zi-Gan-Cao-Shi-Tang*
Gardenia & Soja Combination	*Chih-Tzu-Shih-Tang* *Zhi-Zi-Shi-Tang*
Forsythia & Rhubarb Formula	*Liang-Ke-San* *Liang-Ge-San*
* Gentiana Combination	*Lung-Tan-Hsieh-Kan-Tang* *Long-Dan-Xue-Gan-Tang*
* Ginseng & Gypsum Combination	*Pai-Hu-Chia-Jen-Sheng-Tang* *Bai-Hu-Jia-Ren-Sheng-Tang*
Gypsum Combination	*Pai-Hu-Tang* *Bai-Hu-Tang*
* Lotus Seed Combination	*Ching-Hsin-Lien-Tzu-Yin* *Qing-Xin-Lian-Zi-Yin*
* Magnolia Flower & Gypsum Combination	*Hsin-I-Ching-Fei-Tang* *Xin-I-Qing-Fei-Tang*
* Morus & Lycium Formula	*Hsieh-Pai-San* *Xie-Bai-San*
* Phellodendron Combination	*Tzu-Yin-Chiang-Huo-Tang* *Zi-Yin-Jiang-Huo-Tang*

* Sweet Combination	*Kan-Lu-Yin* *Gan-Lu-Yin*
Rhinoceros & Rehmannia Combination	*Hsi-Chiao-Ti-Huang-Tang* *Xi-Jiao-Di-Huang-Tang*
Saussurea & Coptis Formula	*Hsiang-Lien-Wan* *Xiong-Lian-Wan*
Siler & Licorice Formula	*Hsieh-Huang-San* *Xie-Huang-San*
Anemone Combination	*Pai-Tou-Weng-Tang* *Bai-Tou-Weng-Tang*
Rehmannia & Lonicera Formula	*Pai-Tu-San* *Bai-Tu-San*

Clear Heat

Scute & Cimicifuga Combination	*Pu-Chi-Hsiao-Tu-Yin* *Bu-Qi-Xiao-Tu-Yin*
Scute 3 Herb Combination	*San-Wu-Huang-Chin-Tang* *San-Wu-Huang-Jin-Tang*
Rhubarb Combination	*Ta-Huang-Huang-Lien-Hsieh-Hsin-Tang* *Da-Huang-Huang-Lian-Xie-Xin-Tang*
Rehmannia & Akebia Formula	*Tao-Chih-San* *Tao-Zhi-San*
Xanthium Formula	*Tsang-Erh-San* *Zang-Er-San*
Bupleurum & Pinellia Combination	*Tsing-Fu-Tang* *Zing-Fu-Tang*
Rehmannia & Gypsum Combination	*Yu-Nu-Chien* *Yu-Nu-Chien*

7
Hsiao Tao Chi
(消導劑 , Digestive Formulas)

Formulas that aid digestion and dissolve congestion are called *hsiao tao chi* or *hsiao tao hua chi chi.* The "digestion" method is another of eight Chinese therapeutic methods.

Drinks and foods may injure the stomach, causing nausea, distention, belching with an acidic and fetid odor, and diarrhea. Treatment stimulates digestion and channels the accumulation of undigested food. If there is a conflict between chills, fever, sputum and food and congestion of *ch'i* and blood have resulted in the formation of a hard mass, palpable or non-palpable, treatment focuses on dissolving the hardening and accumulation. Hence, this type of formula is used for conditions due to malfunctioning of the spleen and stomach, for impeded circulation of *ch'i* that results in obstruction and distention, and for movable or non-movable tumors which have developed from the accumulation of moisture, phlegm, food, and blood. Digestive formulas stimulate circulation of *ch'i* and blood and restore normal functioning of the organs.

Both the digestive and the purgative formulas are used to eliminate tangible harmful toxins. However, clinically they are used differently. A purgative formula is indicated for urgent, tangible, harmful toxins whereas a digestive formula is indicated for obstruction, distention, and tumors. A digestive formula treats by means of slowing digestion and moderately dispersing.

Although a digestive formula is milder in action than a purgative, it can be useless or even destructive and is prohibited in weak conformations. Severe accumulation or large growths need to be treated by more potent formulas. A digestive formula might prove too weak and may delay and even hinder recovery. Hence, the practitioner must first weigh the weakness and firmness, consider the harmful toxin and *ch'i,* and recognize the acuteness or chronicity and the mildness or severity of the disease before diagnosing the conformation and prescribing the appropriate formula.

Hsiao Tao Chi
 Shao Tao Qi Dissolve Congestion by "Digestion"

* Hoelen & Alisma Combination	*Fen-Hsiao-Tang* *Fen-Xiao-Tang*
* Magnolia & Ginger Formula	*Ping-Wei-San* *Bing-Wei-San*
Lotus & Citrus Combination	*Chi-Pi-Tang* *Qi-Pi-Tang*
Cyperus & Cluster Combination	*Hsiang-Sha-Yang-Wei-Tang* *Xiong-Sha-Yang-Wei-Tang*
Citrus & Crataegus Formula	*Pao-Ho-Wan* *Bao-Ho-Wan*
Ginseng Stomach Combination	*Jen-Sheng-Yang-Wei-Tang* *Ren-Shen-Yang-Wei-Tang*
Pueraria Flower Combination	*Ko-Hua-Chieh-Hsing-Tang* *Ge-Hua-Jie-Xing-Tang*
Pinellia, Atractylodes, & Agastache Formula	*Pu-Huan-Chin-Cheng-Chi-San* *Ba-Huang-Jin-Jeng-Qi-San*

8
Ching Shu Chi
(清暑劑 , Heat Dispelling Formulas)

Formulas that expel summer toxins and treat summer diseases are called *ching shu chi.*

A heat-dispelling formula acts mainly to dispel "summer toxins," or feverish diseases that occur during summer when the earth is humid and hot. At such times people are subject to the toxins that flourish in heat and moisture and cause illness. Sometimes people cool themselves by lying outdoors without concern for the wind and cool breezes. As a consequence they become chilled. Summer *ch'i,* another summer disease, is connected to the heart, and people with a *ch'i* weakness conformation usually sweat excessively. Hence heat dispelling formulas always include herbs that can dissolve moistness, disperse surface toxins, strengthen *ch'i,* and promote salivation.

Application of the *ching shu chi* is determined by the presence or absence of any accompanying conformation, the chief and subordinate symptoms, and the mildness or seriousness of a summer disease. If a summer disease is accompanied by a "moist condition" such that the disease is serious but fluid retention mild, the "moisture condition" often turns to fever. Thus the formula prescribed should not be too warm and dry or it will dry up the saliva and body fluids. If the fluid retention is more severe and the summer fever mild, the fever often will be masked by the accumulated moisture. If this condition prevails, a sweet and chilly formula should be prescribed.

Ching Shu Chi
Qing Shu Chi Clear Summer Heat Formulas

Astragalus & Atractylodes Combination	*Ching-Shu-I-Chi-Tang* *Qing-Shu-I-Qi-Tang*
Bamboo Leaves & Gypsum Combination	*Chu-Yeh-Shih-Kao-Tang* *Qu-Ye-Shi-Gao-Tang*
Elsholtzia Combination	*Hsiang-Ju-Yin* *Xiong-Ru-Yin*
Elsholtzia Ten Combination	*Shih-Wei-Hsiang-Ju-Yin* *Shi-Wei-Xiong-Ru-Yin*

9
Pu I Chi
(補益劑 , Supplementing Formulas or Tonics)

Formulas that nourish and supplement inadequacy of *ch'i*, blood, yin, and yang are called *pu i chi*. "Supplementing" is one of the eight Chinese therapeutic methods. When the human body is healthy, Chinese physicians say there is a "balance of yin and yang." If either yin or yang is excessive or insufficient, the body is in an abnormal state. A *pu i chi* formula functions to supplement or enrich inadequacy of *ch'i* and blood, to adjust an abundance of yin and yang, and to restore the proper balance. [An ancient saying is, inadequacy is supplemented and surplus is deducted (by these formulas).]

Precautions must be taken in prescribing tonics. Attention must be paid to the phenomenon "strong firmness with weak manifestation" which is a pseudo-weak conformation. This conformation may appear quite similar to a weak and chilly surface conformation, when in fact it is a firm fever accumulated in the interior. If this condition is treated with a tonic formula, it will be aggravated. Cases in which a surface conformation is accompanied by internal weakness or a weak conformation by firmness must be treated with great care. If they are treated with a tonic, a condition likened to "confine the burglar inside the door" may suddenly develop.

Pu I Chi
Bu I Qi Tonify *Qi*/Nourishing *Xue* Formulas, i.e. "Supplementing"

* Anemarrhena, Phellodendron, & Rehmannia Formula	*Chih-Po-Pa-Wei-Wan* *Qie-Po-Ba-Wei-Wan*
* Ginseng & Astragalus Combination	*Pu-Chung-I-Chi-Tang* *Bu-Jung-I-Ji-Tang*
* Ginseng Nutritive Combination	*Jen-Sheng-Yang-Yung-Tang* *Ren-Shen-Yang-Yung-Tang*
* Ginseng & Tang-kuei Formula	*Jen-Sheng-Tang-Shao-San* *Ren-Shen-Tang-Shao-San*

* Ginseng & Tang-kuei 10 Combination	*Shih-Chuan-Ta-Pu-Tang* *Shi-Quan-Da-Pu-Tang*
* Ginseng & Zizyphus Formula	*Tien-Wang-Pu-Hsin-Tan* *Tian-Wang-Bu-Xin-Tan*
* Lycium Formula	*Huan-Shao-Tan* *Huan-Shao-Tan*
* Major 4 Herb Combination	*Szu-Chun-Tzu-Tang* *Si-Jun-Zi-Tang*
* Major 6 Herb Combination	*Liu-Chun-Tzu-Tang* *Liu-Jun-Zi-Tang*
* Pinellia & Ginseng 6 Combination	*Pan-Hsieh-Liu-Chun-Tzu-Tang* *Ban-Xie-Liu-Jun-Zi-Tang*
* Rehmannia 6 Formula	*Liu-Wei-Ti-Huang-Wan* *Liu-Wei-Di-Huang-Wan*
* Rehmannia 8 Formula	*Pa-Wei-Ti-Huang-Wan* *Ba-Wei-Di-Huang-Wan*

_Qi_ "Supplementing Formulas"

* Scute Combination	*Tzu-Sheng-Tung-Erh-Tang* *Zi-Sheng-Tong-Er-Tang*
* Tang-kuei & Ginseng 8 Combination	*Pa Chen-Tang* *Ba-Chen-Tang*
B.P. & Major 6 Herb Combination	*Chai-Shao-Liu-Chun-Tzu-Tang* *Chai-Shao-Liu-Jun-Zi-Tang*
Rehmannia & Schizandra Combination	*Chi-Wei-Tu-Chi-Wan* *Qi-Wei-Tu-Qi-Wan*
Siler & Chiang-huo Combination	*Chia-Wei-Pa-Hsien-Tang* *Jia-Wei-Ba-Xian-Tang*
Atractylodes & Pueraria Formula	*Chien-Shih-Pai-Chu-San* *Jian-Shi-Bai-Ju-San*
Chin-chiu & Bupleurum Combination	*Chin-Chiu-Fu-Lei-Tang* *Jin-Ju-Fu-Lei-Tang*
Chin-chiu & Tortoise Shell Formula	*Chin-Chiu-Pieh-Chia-San* *Jin-Ju-Bia-Jia-San*
Saussurea & Cardamon Combination	*Hsiang-Sha-Liu-Chun-Tzu-Tang* *Xiong-Sha-Liu-Jun-Zi-Tang*
Astragalus & Cinnamon 5 Herb Combination	*Huang-Chi-Kuei-Chih-Wu-Wu-Tang* *Huang-Qi-Gui-Zhi-Wu-Wu-Tang*

Astragalus & Tortoise Shell Formula	*Huang-Chi-Pieh-Chia-San* *Huang-Qi-Pie-Jia-San*
Ginseng, Astragalus, & Pueraria Combination	*I-Chi-Chung-Ming-Tang* *I-Qi-Jung-Ming-Tang*
Achyranthes & Plantago Formula	*Niu-Che-Shen-Chi-Wan* *Niu-Che-Shen-Chi-Wan*
Lily Combination	*Pai-Ho-Ku-Chin-Tang* *Bai-He-Gu-Jin-Tang*
Gelatin & Aristolochia Combination	*Pu-Fei-Ah-Chiao-Tang* *Bu-Fei-E-Jiao-Tang*
Tang-kuei & Rehmannia Combination	*Pu-Yin-Tang* *Bu-Yin-Tang*
Dioscorea Combination	*Szu-Shen-Tang* *Si-Shen-Tang*
Tang-kuei & Astragalus Combination	*Tang-kuei-Pu-Hsieh-Tang* *Dang-Gui-Bu-Xue-Tang*
Tang-kuei, Ginger, & Mutton Combination	*Tang-Kuei-Sheng-Chiang-Yang-Zou-Tang* *Dang-Gui-Sheng-Qiang-Yang-Zou-Tang*
Loadstone & Rehmannia Formula	*Tsu-Shih-Ti-Huang-Wan* *Zi-Shi-Di-Huang-Wan*
Aster Combination	*Tzu-Wan-Tang* *Zi-Wan-Tang*
Eucommia & Achyranthes Formula	*Wei-Cheng-Fang* *Wei-Cheng-Fang*
Astragalus & Zizyphus Combination	*Yang-Hsin-Tang* *Yang-Xin-Tang*

10
Chu Han Chi
(祛寒劑 , Chill Dispelling Formulas)

Formulas composed chiefly of warm- or hot-natured herbs intended to dispel "stale chills" residing in the viscera are called *chu han chi.*

The *chu han chi* treat a degenerated yang *ch'i* when yin chills are thriving internally. Ancient proverbs say to "heat chills," or "treat chills with hot herbs." Thus the rule of treatment for dispelling chills.

Interior chills are due to a yang deficiency, or to external chills that have invaded the interior, or to an injury of yang *ch'i* as a consequence of taking the wrong medication. Therefore, formulas recorded in this section are divided into two types: interior-warming, chill-dispelling formulas and yang-restoring, chill-curing formulas.

A fever lying dormant internally causes chills and the stronger the fever, the more severe the chills. This condition is one of internal real fever and external pseudo-chills. The doctor after carefully analyzing and diagnosing this condition should not prescribe a warm or hot formula. Dosages must vary according to the individual's condition. For persons with a thriving fever or an injured yin from loss of blood, the dose should be kept small even if the patient has a chill conformation that calls for a warm formula. As soon as the formula has taken effect, it should be suspended so that it will not affect the patient's physique and induce unnecessary changes.

Chu Han Chi
Qu Han Qi Dispel Cold by Warming the Interior Formulas

* Aconite & G. L. Combination	*Szu-Ni-Tang* *Si-Ni-Tang*
* Astragalus Combination	*Huang-Chi-Chien-Chung-Tang* *Huang-Qi-Jian-Zhong-Tang*
Atractylodes & Aconite Combination	*Pai-Chu-Fu-Tzu-Tang* *Bai-Zhi-Fu-Zi-Tang*
* Cinnamon, Aconite, & Ginger Combination	*Kuei-Chih-Fu-Tzu-Tang* *Gui-Zhi-Fu-Zi-Tang*

* Cinnamon & Atractylodes Combination	*Kuei-Chih-Chia-Ling-Chu-Fu-Tang* *Gui-Zhi-Jia-Ling-Qu-Fu-Tang*
* Cinnamon & Ginseng Combination	*Kuei-Chih-Jen-Sheng-Tang* *Gui-Zhi-Ren-Shen-Tang*
* Evodia Combination	*Wu-Chu-Yu-Tang* *Wu-Chu-Yu-Tang*
* Ginseng & Ginger Combination	*Jen-Sheng-Tang/Li-Chung-Tang* *Ren-Shen-Tang/Li-Zhong-Tang*
* Licorice & Aconite Combination	*Kan-Tsao-Fu-Tzu-Tang* *Gan-Cao-Fu-Zi-Tang*
* Licorice & Ginger Combination	*Kan-Tsao-Kan-Chiang-Tang* *Gan-Cao-Gan-Jiang-Tang*
* Major Zanthoxylum Combination	*Ta-Chien-Chung-Tang* *Da-Jian-Zhong-Tang*
* Minor Cinnamon & Peony Combination	*Hsiao-Chien-Chung-Tang* *Shao-Jian-Zhong-Tang*
* Tang-kuei, Evodia, & Ginger Combination	*Tang-Kuei-Szu-Ni-Chia-Wu-Chu-Yu-Sheng-Chiang-Tang* *Dang-Gui-Si-Ni-Jia-Wu-Chu-Yu-Sheng-Jiang-Tang*
* Vitality Combination	*Chen-Wu-Tang* *Chen-Wu-Tang*
Zanthoxylum Combination	*Chieh-Chi-Shu-Chiao-Tang* *Qie-Ji-Shu-Qiao-Tang*
Tang-kuei Combination	*Chien-Chin-Tang-Kuei-Tang* *Jian-Jiu-Dang-Gui-Tang*
Hoelen, G. L. & Aconite Combination	*Fu-Ling-Szu-Ni-Tang* *Fu-Ling-Si-Ni-Tang*
Aconite & Oryza Combination	*Fu-Tzu-Keng-Mi-Tang* *Fu-Zi-Geng-Mi-Tang*
Aconite, Ginseng, & Ginger Combination	*Fu-Tzu-Li-Chung-Tang* *Fu-Si-Li-Zhong-Tang*
Aconite Combination	*Fu-Tzu-Tang* *Fu-Zi-Tang*
Magnolia & Saussurea Combination	*Hou-Pu-Wen-Chung-Tang* *Hou-Po-Wen-Zhong-Tang*
Peony, Licorice, & Aconite Combination	*Shao-Yao-Kan-Tsao-Fu-Tzu-Tang* *Shao-Yao-Gan-Cao-Fu-Zi-Tang*

G.L. & Aconite Combination w̄ ginseng	*Szu-Ni-Chia-Jen-Sheng-Tang* *Si-Ni-Jia-Ren-Shen-Tang*
Tang-kuei, Cinnamon, & Peony Combination	*Tang-Kuei-Chien-Chung-Tang* *Dang-Gui-Jian-Zhong-Tang*
Tang-kuei & Jujube Combination	*Tang-Kuei-Szu-Ni-Tang* *Dang-Gui-Si-Ni-Tang*
Licorice, Aconite, & Ginger Pulse Combination	*Tung-Mo-Szu-Ni-Tang* *Tong-Mo-Si-Ni-Tang*
Wu-tou & Cinnamon Combination	*Wu-Tou-Kuei-Chih-Tang* *Wu-Tou-Gui-Zhi-Tang*

11
Kai Chiao Tung Kuan Chi
(開竅通關劑 , Smelling Salts, Inhalants)

Formulas composed chiefly of aromatic and "penetrative" herbs treat unconsciousness or a coma and are called *kai chiao tung kuan chi* or *fang hsiang kai kung chi.*

Unconsciousness and comas are differentiated into heat and chill closure. Accordingly, in clinical practice, the formulas are also divided into cool and warm. Cool-opening formulas are composed of aromatic herbs together with fever reducing and detoxicant herbs or with blood cooling and antispasmodic herbs. The formulas cleanse the heart, relieve faintness, lower fevers, and detoxify. The herbal formulas used in the warm-opening method are composed of aromatic herbs together with acrid, warm, *ch'i*-moving, and obstruction-dissolving herbs. They awaken the patient and dissolve turbidity by means of the smell of the herbs.

Before using smelling salts, the doctor must determine whether the conformation is chilly or hot; whereupon the decision to use a cool or warm formula can be made. Moreover, no matter which awakening method, this type of formula is only suitable for an "obstruction conformation" in which harmful toxin is thriving and the patient's *ch'i* is full. Unconscious patients with toneless hands, incontinence, feeble and minute respiration, and spontaneous perspiration – a "prostration" conformation – cannot be treated with these formulas even in the presence of delirium and coma.

Kai Chiao Tung Kuan Chi
Gai Jiao Tong Guan Qi Smelling Salts for Resuscitation

Bos & Curcuma Formula	*An-Kung-Niu-Huang-Wan* *An-Gung-Niu-Huang-Wan*
Rhinoceros & Succinum Formula	*Chih-Pao-Tan* *Zhi-Bao-Tan*
Bos & Musk Formula	*Niu-Huang-Ching-Hsin-Wan* *Niu-Huang-Ching-Hsin-Wan*

Styrax Formula	*Su-Ho-Hsiang-Wan* *Su-Ho-Hsiang-Wan*
Gleditsia & Asarum Formula	*Tung-Kuan-San* *Tong-Guan-San*
Rhinoceros & Antelope Horn Formula	*Tzù-Hsueh-Tan* *Zi-Xue-Tan*

12
Chen Ching Chi
(鎮靜劑 , Sedative Formulas)

Formulas with sedative and tranquilizing effects are called *chen ching chi.* A *chen ching chi* formula reduces pain, arrests spasms, and quiets hysteria. According to origin, pathological mechanism, and herbal action, *chen ching chi* are divided into strong, sedating tranquilizers and heart-nourishing, mind sedatives. The former contains mostly heavy minerals and stones or shells that calm hysteria and tranquilize the mind by means of their heaviness; the latter is composed mainly of herbs that nourish the heart and pacify the mind while enriching the liver.

Because minerals, stones, and shells are detrimental to the spleen and stomach, strong tranquilizers should be used only temporarily.

Chen Ching Chi
Chen Jing Qi Sedative Formulas

* Bupleurum Formula	*I-Kan-San* *I-Gan-San*
* Bupleurum & Dragon Bone Combination	*Chai-Hu-Chia-Lung-Ku-Mu-Li-Tang* *Chai-Hu-Jia-Long-Gu-Mu-Li-Tang*
* Cinnamon & Dragon Bone Combination	*Kuei-Chih-Chia-Lung-Ku-Mu-Li-Tang* *Gui-Zhi-Jia-Long-Gu-Mu-Li-Tang*
* Licorice Combination	*Kan-Tsao-Tang* *Gan-Cao-Tang*
* Licorice & Jujube Combination	*Kan-Mai-Ta-Tsao-Tang* *Gan-Mai-Da-Zao-Tang*
* Zizyphus Combination	*Suan-Tsao-Jen-Tang* *Suan-Zao-Ren-Tang*
Cinnabar Formula	*Chu-Sha-An-Shen-Wan* *Qu-Sha-An-Shen-Wan*

Bupleurum & Citrus, Pinellia Formula	*I-Kan-San-Chia-Chen-Pi-Pan-Hsia* *I-Gan-San-Jia-Chen-Pi-Ban-Xia*
Cinnamon & D.D.O. Combination	*Kuei-Chih-Chu-Shao-Yao-Chia-Shu-Chi-Lung-Ku-Mu-Li-Tang* *Gui-Zhi-Ju-Sha-Yao-Jia-Shu-Chi-Long-Gu-Mu-Li-Tang*
Dragon Bone & Oyster Shell Combination	*Lung-Ku-Mu-Li-Tang* *Long-Gu-Mu-Li-Tang*

13
Sho She Chi
(收濇劑 , Astringent Formulas)

Formulas composed mainly of astringent and restraining herbs that treat loss, debilitation, wasting, and exhaustion of *ch'i,* blood, or sperm are called *sho she chi.*

An astringent formula is principally used for spontaneous sweating, night sweats, a prolonged cough, mild asthma, chronic diarrhea, spermatorrhea, urinary incontinence, uterine hemorrhage, uterine discharge, and hemorrhoidal bleeding. The classics say: "If there is looseness, we astringe it, and astringency restrains prolapses."

These formulas arrest sweating, coughing, excessive menstrual flow and leukorrhea; tone the skin and muscle and thus restrain prolapses; astringe the lungs and intestines; and stimulate sperm production. They are contraindicated in the presence of fever with hyperhidrosis, sputum stagnancy with asthmatic cough, initial feverish diarrhea, diarrhea due to tainted food, and "fire agitation" that causes spermatorrhea.

Sho She Chi
Sho She Qi Astringent-restraining Formulas

* Lotus Stamen Formula	*Chin-Sou-Ku-Ching-Wan* *Qin-Sou-Gu-Jing-Wan*
Hoelen & Polyporus Formula	*Chih-Cho-Ku-Pen-Wan* *Zhi-Zhou-Gu-Ben-Wan*
Kaolin & Limonite Combination	*Chih-Shih-Chih-Yu-Yu-Liang-Tang* *Zhi-Shi-Zhi-Yu-Yu-Liang-Tang*
Hoelen & Cuscuta Formula	*Fu-Tu-Tan* *Fu-Tu-Tan*
Mantis Formula	*Sang-Piao-Hsiao-San* *Sang-Biao-Xiao-San*
Kaolin & Oryza Combination	*Tao-Hua-Tang* *Tao-Hua-Tang*

14
Li Ch'i Chi
(理氣劑 , *Ch'i* Formulas)

Formuas that balance *ch'i* and treat all *ch'i* diseases are termed *ch'i* formulas. *The Yellow Emperor's Classic of Internal Medicine* (黃帝內經) says: "Anger causes an up-rising of *ch'i*, pleasure mollifies *ch'i*, sorrow makes *ch'i* subside, horror makes *ch'i* descend, chills make *ch'i* shrink, fever exhausts *ch'i*, astonishment disturbs *ch'i*, weariness wastes *ch'i*, and worrying obstructs *ch'i*." These nine variations of *ch'i* disturbance give rise to all manner of diseases. Accordingly, the methods to treat *ch'i* diseases vary. For example, a loss or subsidence of *ch'i* must be replenished; an obstruction to *ch'i* must be removed or *ch'i* circulated, and an adversity in *ch'i* must be descended. Clinically there are many ways to treat *ch'i* disorders. These include nourishment and replenishment, discharge and guidance, purgation, expectoration, astringement, and stimulation of blood circulation. Most illnesses cannot be effectively treated without the inclusion of *ch'i* herbs.

When using *ch'i* formulas, the physician has to determine whether the conformation is weak or firm. If the condition calls for supplementation and *ch'i* moving herbs are used instead, *ch'i* will become weaker and empty. If the condition requires circulating *ch'i* but *ch'i* tonics are used instead, the *ch'i* will become further stagnated. If it is a complex condition, so that there is a trace of weakness within firmness, then *ch'i* supplementing and *ch'i*-moving formulas are used concomitantly. Because most *ch'i* formulas contain herbs that are aromatic, arid, bitter, and warm, *ch'i* obstruction accompanied with fluid deficiency and injury is treated deliberately.

Li Ch'i Chi
Li Qi Ji *Qi* Formulas

* Areca & Evodia Combination	*Pien-Chih-Hsin-Chi-Yin* *Bian-Zhi-Xin-Ji-Yin*
* Cardamon & Fennel Formula	*An-Chung-San* *An-Zhong-San*

* Gambir Formula	*Kou-Teng-San* *Kon-Teng-San*
* Inula & Hematite Combination	*Hsuan-Fu-Hua-Tai-Che-Shih-Tang* *Xuan-Fu-Hua-Tai-Che-Shi-Tang*
* Lindera Formula	*Wu-Yao-Shun-Chi-San* *Wu-Yao-Shun-Ji-San*
* Mahuang & Ginkgo Combination	*Ting-Chuan-Tang* *Ding-Chuan-Tang*
* Perilla Fruit Combination	*Su-Tzu-Chiang-Chi-Tang* *Su-Zi-Xiang-Ji-Tang*

***Qi* Formulas**

* Pinellia & Magnolia Combination	*Pan-Hsia-Hou-Pu-Tang* *Ban-Xia-Hou-Po-Tang*
* Mahuang & Magnolia Combination	*Shen-Mi-Tang* *Shen-Mi-Tang*
Lindera & Cyperus Formula	*Chen-Chi-Tien-Hsiang-San* *Chen-Ji-Tian-Xiang-San*
Aquilaria & Gastrodia Combination	*Chen-Hsiang-Tien-Ma-Tang* *Chen-Xiang-Tian-Ma-Tang*
Chih-shih, Bakeri, & Cinnamon Combination	*Chih-Shih-Hsieh-Pai-Kuei-Chih-Tang* *Zhi-Shi-Xie-Bai-Gui-Zhi-Tang*
Aurantium & Bamboo Combination	*Chu-Pi-Chu-Ju-Tang* *Ju-Pi-Gu-Ru-Tang*
Atractylodes & Cardamon Combination	*Chuan-Szu-Chun-Tzu-Tang* *Quan-Si-Zhun-Zi-Tang*
Citrus & Perilla Combination	*Fen-Hsin-Chi-Yin* *Fen-Xin-Ji-Yin*
Magnolia Three Combination	*Hou-Pu-San-Wu-Tang* *Hou-Pu-San-Wu-Tang*
Magnolia Five Combination	*Hou-Pu-Sheng-Chiang-Pan-Hsia-Kan-Tsao-Jen-Sheng-Tang* *Hou-Po-Sheng-Xiang-Ban-Xia-Gan-Cao-Ren-Sheng-Tang*
Cyperus, Perilla, & Citrus Formula	*Hsing-Chi-Hsiang-Su-San* *Xing-Zhi-Xiang-Su-San*
G.P. & Ginseng Formula	*Kan-Chiang-Jen-Sheng-Pan-Hsia-Wan* *Gan-Xiang-Ren-Shen-Ban-Xia-Wan*

Trichosanthes, Bakeri, & Vinegar Combination	*Kua-Lou-Hsieh-Pai-Pai-Chiu-Tang* *Gua-Lou-Xie-Bai-Bai-Qiu-Tang*
Galanga & Chih-shih Combination	*Liang-Chih-Tang* *Liang-Zhi-Tang*
Tang-kuei & Cyperus Formula	*Nu-Shen-San* *Nu-Shen-San*
Aquilaria & Perilla Formula	*San-Ho-San* *San-Ho-San*
Tang-kuei 16 Herb Combination	*Shih-Liu-Wei-Liu-Chi-Yin* *Shi-Liu-Wei-Liu-Ji-Yin*
Kaki Combination	*Shih-Ti-Tang* *Shi-Di-Tang*
Clove & Kaki Combination	*Ting-Hsiang-Shih-Ti-Tang* *Ding-Xiang-Shi-Di-Tang*
Evodia & Pinellia Combination	*Yen-Nien-Pan-Hsia-Tang* *Yen-Nien-Ban-Xia-Tang*

15
Li Hsieh Chi
(理血劑 , Blood Formulas)

Formulas that circulate the blood and treat blood diseases are termed *li hsieh chi.*

The blood carries the nutrients to all parts of the body. An ancient adage says: "When the blood is weak, the body deteriorates, but with healthy blood the eyes can see, the ears can hear, the palms can grip, and the feet can walk." Blood formulas treat poor circulation, occlusion or stagnancy, extravasation and the consequent hemoptysis (hemorrhage of the larynx, trachea, bronchi, or lungs), hematemesis (vomiting blood), hematuria (bloody urine), and bloody feces. The contents of a blood formula varies according to its action. Blood formulas can be divided into hematinic (increasing hemoglobin), hemostatic (stopping bleeding), cooling, and warming types. The hematinic and cooling types are discussed in the sections on *pu yang chi* (補養劑) and *ching je chi* (清熱劑). Here the hemostatic and deobstruent formulas are introduced.

This type of formula belongs to the "attacking" type and should not be used excessively, otherwise *ch'i* will be injured. "Blood flowing within the vessels" is the normal condition. Pathological changes sometimes cause the blood to overflow or pool, resulting in hemorrhage, nosebleeds, bloody urine, or bloody feces. Each condition must be treated with the proper formula with respect to whether the condition is chills, fever, weakness, or firmness: for example, an acute condition uses the palliative hemostasis method; a firm fever calls for a hemostatic as well as a fever-reducing formula; and a weak chill conformation needs a hemostatic formula together with a yang-warming formula. Both the principal and subordinate symptoms have to be noted before a correct treatment can be prescribed.

Li Hsieh Chi
Li Xue Qi Blood Tonics, Circulation and Hemostasis Formulas

* Cinnamon & Hoelen Formula — *Kuei-Chih-Fu-Ling-Wan*
Gui-Zhi-Fu-Ling-Wan

* Clematis & Stephania Combination	*Shu-Ching-Huo-Hsieh-Tang* *Shu-Jing-Huo-Xie-Tang*
* Ginseng & Longan Combination	*Kuei-Pi-Tang* *Gui-Pi-Tang*
* Musk & Catechu Formula	*Chi-Li-San* *Ji-Li-San*
* Persica & Rhubarb Combination	*Tao-Ho-Cheng-Chi-Tang* *Tao-Ho-Zheng-Ji-Tang*
* Tang-kuei 4 Combination	*Szu-Wu-Tang* *Si-Wu-Tang*
* Tang-kuei & Gambir Combination	*Chi-Wu-Chiang-Hsia-Tang* *Ji-Wu-Xiang-Xia-Tang*
* Tang-kuei & Gardenia Combination	*Wen-Ching-Yin* *Wen-Jing-Yin*
Ginseng, Longan, & Bupleurum Combination	*Chia-Wei-Kuei-Pi-Tang* *Jia-Wei-Gui-Pi-Tang*
Gelatin & Artemisia Four Combination	*Chiao-Ai-Szu-Wu-Tang* *Jiao-Ai-Si-Wu-Tang*
Tang-kuei & Persica Combination	*Fu-Yuan-Huo-Hsieh-Tang* *Fu-Yuan-Huo-Xie-Tang*
Fu-lung-kan Combination	*Huang-Tu-Tang* *Huang-Tu-Tang*
Pueraria & Carthamus Combination	*Ko-Ken-Hung-Hua-Tang* *Ge-Gen-Hong-Hua-Tang*
Tang-kuei & Atractylodes Combination	*Lien-Chu-Yin* *Lian-Gu-Yin*
Peony Combination	*Shao-Yao-Tang* *Shao-Yao-Tang*
Bupleurum & Evodia Combination	*Shu-Kan-Tang* *Shu-Gan-Tang*
Rhubarb & Leech Combination	*Ti-Tang-Tang* *Ti-Tang-Tang*
Tang-kuei & Carthamus Formula	*Tung-Tao-San* *Tung-Tao-San*

16
Chu Feng Chi
(祛風劑 , Carminative Formulas)

Formulas that treat all kinds of wind diseases are *chu feng chi.* Wind diseases are broad in scope, the variation in disease condition being very complex. Wind diseases are divided into two major categories: internal and external. Whereas external wind is caused by the six excesses that invade the body and lodge in the meridians, muscles, sinews, and bones, internal wind develops from weakness and deficiency in blood, or from excessive thriving of a harmful fever toxin that causes disorders in circulation of *ch'i* and blood.

The rule of thumb for treatment of external wind diseases is that they are dispersed with acrid and arid herbs. The formulas prescribed must also contain blood nourishing and activating herbs in order to subjugate the strong aridity of such herbs. Internal wind diseases should not be treated with dispersing herbs but with cool and moistening or lubricating herbs. However, if moistening herbs are used in excess, they may hinder the stomach's function. Therefore, every aspect of a patient's condition must be considered before prescribing a formula.

Chu Feng Chi
Zhu Feng Qi Wind-dispelling Carminative Formulas

* Cinnamon & Anemarrhena Combination	*Kuei-Chih-Shao-Yao-Chih-Mu-Tang* *Gui-Zhi-Shao-Yao-Zhi-Mu-Tang*
* Clematis & Carthamus Formula	*Shu-Chin-Li-An-San* *Shu-Jin-Li-An-San*
* Major Siler Combination	*Ta-Fang-Feng-Tang* *Da-Fang-Feng-Tang*
* Mahuang & Ginseng Combination	*Hsu-Ming-Tang* *Xu-Ming-Tang*
* Tang-kuei & Arctium Formula	*Hsiao-Feng-San* *Hsiao-Feng-San*

* Tu-huo & Vaeicum Combination	*Tu-Huo-Chi-Sheng-Tang* *Tu-Huo-Ji-Sheng-Tang*
Ophiopogon & Asarum Combination	*Ching-Shang-Chuan-Tung-Tang* *Jing-Shang-Quan-Tong-Tang*
Chiang-huo & Tumeric Combination	*Chuan-Pi-Tang* *Quan-Pi-Tang*
Mahuang & Peony Combination	*Hsiao-Hsu-Ming-Tang* *Shao-Xu-Ming-Tang*
Cinnamon & Angelica Formula	*Shang-Chung-Hsia-Tung-Yung-Tung-Feng-Wan* *Shang-Zhong-Xia-Tong-Yong-Tong-Feng-Wan*
Astragalus & Aconite Formula	*Shih-Wei-Tsuo-San* *Shih-Wei-Zou-San*
Stephania & Carthamus Combination	*Shu-Feng-Huo-Hsieh-Tang* *Shu-Feng-Huo-Xu-Tang*
Atractylodes & Setaria Combination	*Wei-Feng-Tang* *Wei-Feng-Tang*

17
Chu Shih Chi
(祛濕劑 , Diuretics)

Formulas that treat body fluids are called *chu shih chi.*

Fluids are either yin chilly, heavily turbid, or sticky and poisonous. They are divided into internal and external fluids, or water. Internal fluids are further differentiated into upper, middle, and the lower. The fluid may also be affected by the fever toxin generated by wind, chills, heat, and fever. Therapeutically the location of the toxin is determined and treate accordingly. Diuretics increase water flow and discharge, relieve urinary stuttering, and bring about the excretion. Depending on whether the condition is humid and warm, formulas are prescribed according to the presence of diarrhea, dysentery, edema, or jaundice.

In treating a water conformation, attention must be given to a yin-weakness or saliva drying-up conformation for which a diuretic formula is contraindicated. Because a diuretic will dry salivation, it is necessary to incorporate other herbs. This is especially true for bitter and arid herbs which should be used with extreme care. For example, post-illness edema due to splenic weakness or foot edema in pregnant women are conditions calling for diuresis, but the prescription must incorporate spleen-strengthening tonics in order to protect *ch'i.*

Chu Shih Chi
Zhu Shi Qi Diuretic Formulas

* Alisma Combination	*Tse-Hsieh-Tang* *Ze-Xie-Tang*
* Areca Seed Combination	*Chiu-Ping-Wu-Fu-Tang* *Qiu-Bing-Wu-Fu-Tang*
* Atractylodes Combination	*Yueh-Pi-Chia-Chu-Tang* *Yue-Pi-Jiu-Zhu-Tang*
* Atractylodes & Hoelen Combination	*Ling-Kuei-Chu-Kan-Tang* *Ling-Gui-Chu-Gan-Tang*

* Bupleurum & Hoelen Combination	*Chai-Ling-Tang* *Chai-Ling-Tang*
* Capillaris Combination	*Yin-Chen-Hao-Tang* *Yin-Chen-Hao-Tang*
* Capillaris & Hoelen Formula	*Yin-Chen-Wu-Ling-San* *Yin-Chen-Wu-Ling-San*
* Coix Combination	*I-Yi-Jen-Tang* *I-Yi-Ren-Tang*
* Dianthus Formula	*Pa-Cheng-San* *Ba-Zheng-San*
* Hoelen Five Herb Formula	*Wu-Ling-San* *Wu-Ling-San*
* Magnolia & Hoelen Combination	*Wei-Ling-Tang* *Wei-Ling-Tang*
* Minor Pinellia & Hoelen Combination	*Hsiao-Pan-Hsia-Chia-Fu-Ling-Tang* *Shao-Ban-Xia-Jia-Fu-Ling-Tang*
* Stephania & Astragalus Combination	*Fang-Chi-Huang-Chi-Tang* *Fang-Qi-Huang-Qi-Tang*

Diuretics

* Stephania & Ginseng Combination	*Mu-Fang-Chi-Tang* *Mu-Fang-Qi-Tang*
* Tang-kuei & Anemarrhena Combination	*Tang-Kuei-Nien-Tung-Tang* *Dang-Gui-Lian-Tong-Tang*
Areca Seed & Chaenomeles Formula	*Chi-Ming-San* *Ji-Ming-San*
Hoelen & Jujube Combination	*Chien-Chung-Tang* *Jian-Zhong-Tang*
Gardenia & Phellodendron Combination	*Chih-Tzu-Po-Pi-Tang* *Zhi-Zi-Bo-Pe-Tang*
Polyporus Combination	*Chu-Ling-Tang* *Zhu-Ling-Tang*
Atractylodes & Arisaema Combination	*Erh-Chu-Tang* *Er-Zhu-Tang*
Stephania & Hoelen Combination	*Fang-Chi-Fu-Ling-Tang* *Fang-Qi-Fu-Ling-Tang*
Licorice & Hoelen Combination	*Fu-Ling-Kan-Tsao-Tang* *Fu-Ling-Gan-Cao-Tang*

Alisma & Hoelen Combination	*Fu-Ling-Tse-Hsieh-Tang* *Fu-Ling-Ze-Xie-Tang*
Hoelen Combination	*Fu-Ling-Yin* *Fu-Ling-Yin*
Ginger & Hoelen Combination	*Ling-Chiang-Chu-Kan-Tang* *Ling-Xiang-Zhu-Gan-Tang*
Hoelen, Licorice, & Jujube Combination	*Ling-Kuei-Kan-Tsao-Tang* *Ling-Gui-Gan-Cao-Tang*
Hoelen, Licorice, & Schizandra Combination	*Ling-Kuei-Wei-Kan-Tang* *Ling-Gui-Wei-Gan-Tang*
Mahuang, Forsythia, & Phaseolus Combination	*Ma-Huang-Lien-Chiao-Chih-Hsiao-Tou-Tang* *Ma-Huang-Lian-Jiao-Zhi-Xiao-Tou-Tang*
Hoelen & Akebia Combination	*Mi-Niao-Chien* *Mi-Niao-Jian*
Tokoro Combination	*Pi-Hsieh-Fen-Ching-Yin* *Bi-Xie-Fen-Zhong-Yin*
Magnolia & Atractylodes Combination	*Shih-Pi-Yin* *Shi-Pi-Yin*
Hoelen, Atractylodes, & Areca Combination	*Tao-Shui-Fu-Ling-Tang* *Dao-Shui-Fu-Ling-Tang*
Clove & Hoelen Combination	*Ting-Hsiang-Fu-Ling-Tang* *Ting-Xiong-Fu-Ling-Tang*
Hoelen & Areca Combination	*Wu-Pi-Yin* *Wu-Pi-Yin*
Mahuang, Gypsum, & Pinellia Combination	*Yueh-Pi-Chia-Pan-Hsia-Tang* *Yueh-Bi-Jia-Ban-Xia-Tang*
Mahuang & Gypsum Combination	*Yueh-Pi-Tang* *Yueh-Pi-Tang*

18
Jun Tsao Chi
(潤燥劑 , Moistening Formulas)

Formulas using nourishing and moistening herbs to treat an arid conformation (dehydration) are termed *jun tsao chi.*

An arid conformation is either internal or external. External aridity occurs during the autumn. Since the autumn weather may be warm or cool, a contracted harmful toxin will manifest itself in either warm or cool conformations. Internal aridity is also either cool or warm. It is due to exhaustion and a lack of visceral fluids, and depending on the location of illness, it is further divided into upper, middle, and lower aridity. Treatment for an arid conformation includes either moistening the aridity with light herbs dispersing herbs or moistening the aridity with sweet and chilly herbs.

Obviously both acrid, aromatic herbs that exhaust saliva and bitter, chilly herbs that harm *ch'i* are contraindicated for aridity diseases.

Jun Tsao Chi
Run Cao Qi Moistening/emollient formulas to counter dehydration

* Apricot Seed & Linum Formula	*Ma-Tzu-Jen-Wan* *Ma-Zi-Ren-Wan*
* Eriobotrya & Ophiopogon Combination	*Ching-Tsao-Chiu-Fei-Tang* *Jing-Cao-Jiu-Fei-Tang*
* Linum & Rhubarb Combination	*Jun-Chang-Tang* *Run-Chang-Tang*
* Ophiopogon Combination	*Mai-Men-Tung-Tang* *Mai-Men-Tong-Tang*
Baked Licorice Combination	*Chih-Kan-Tsao-Tang* *Zhi-Gan-Cao-Tang*
Cnidium & Moutan Combination	*Ching-Je-Pu-Hsieh-Tang* *Jing-Re-Bu-Xue-Tang*

Ophiopogon & Trichosanthes Combination	*Mai-Men-Tung-Yin-Tzu* *Mai-Men-Tong-Yin-Zi*
Tang-kuei & Tribulus Combination	*Tang-Kuei-Yin-Tzu* *Dang-Gui-Yin-Zi*

19
Chu Tan Chi
(除痰劑, Expectorant Formulas)

Formulas that help expel or eliminate excessive sputum (mucus) and saliva are termed expectorant formulas.

Sputum is either wet, dry, hot, chilly, or "windy." Substantially sputum and saliva are composed of water and so are also known as "water toxin." Water toxin results from a functional disturbance in the spleen and kidneys, but most commonly in the spleen. Hence, most expectorants are spleen-healing formulas.

Excessive mucus or saliva either tickles or blocks the trachea, causing a cough and an increase in the generation and secretion of sputum.

Therefore, therapeutically an expectorant is often combined with a cough suppressant in order to bring about a favorable effect.

Chu Tan Chi
Zhu Dan Qi Expectorants

* Bupleurum & Scute Combination	*Chai-Hsien-Tang* *Chai-Xian-Tang*
* Gasping Formula	*Hsiang-Sheng-Po-Ti-Wan* *Xiong-Sheng-Bo-Di-Wan*
* Hoelen & Schizandra Combination	*Ling-Kan-Chiang-Wei-Hsin-Hsia-Jen-Tang* *Ling-Gan-Xiong-Wei-Xin-Xia-Ren-Tang*
* Pinellia & Gardenia Combination	*Li-Ke-Tang* *Le-Ge-Tang*
* Pinellia & Gastrodia Combination	*Pan-Hsia-Pai-Chu-Tien-Ma-Tang* *Ban-Xia-Bai-Zhi-Tian-Ma-Tang*
Morus & Platycodon Formula	*Tun-Sou-San* *Tun-Sou-San*
Platycodon & Schizonepeta Formula	*Chih-Sou-San* *Zhi-Sou-San*

Schizonepeta & Pinellia Formula	*Chin-Fei-Tsao-San* *Jin-Fei-Cao-San*
Pinellia & Arisaema Combination	*Ching-Shih-Hua-Tan-Tang* *Jing-Shi-Hua-Dan-Tang*
Citrus & Pinellia Combination	*Erh-Chen-Tang* *Er-Chen-Tang*
Trichosanthes & Chih-shih Combination	*Kua-Lou-Chih-Shih-Tang* *Gua-Lou-Zhi-Shi-Tang*
Lapis & Scute Formula	*Meng-Shih-Kuen-Tan-Wan* *Meng-Shi-Guen-Tan-Wan*
Fritillary & Platycodon Formula	*Ning-Sou-Wan* *Ning-Sou-Wan*

20
Chu Chung Chi
(驅蟲劑 , Anthelmintic Formulas)

Formulas that dispel parasitic worms are named *chu chung chi.*

An anthelmintic either dispels or kills parasitic worms living in the alimentary tract. People suffering from parasites often have a swollen and aching belly; loss of appetite or a voracious appetite, often favoring peculiar foods; and irregular bowel movements. As the condition continues the patient may become withered and yellow and emaciated. Depending on the type of parasites, anthelmintics are classified as ascaricide, (agent that kills nematodes), taeniacide (agent that kills tapeworms), oxyuricide (agent that kills pinworms), and ankylostomiacide (agent that kills hookworms).

Chu Chung Chi
Zhu Zhang Qi Anthelmintic Formulas

Licorice, Minium, & Honey Combination	*Kan-Tsao-Fen-Mi-Tang* *Gan-Cao-Fen-Mi-Tang*
Ginseng & Zanthoxylum Combination	*Li-Chung-An-Huei-Tang* *Li-Chung-An-Huei-Tang*
Picrorrhiza & Mume Combination	*Lien-Mei-An-Huei-Tang* *Lian-Mei-An-Huei-Tang*
Mume Formula	*Wu-Mei-Wan* *Wu-Mei-Wan*

21
Ching Chan Chi
(經產劑 , Gyneco-obstetric Formulas)

Formulas for women that treat abnormal menstruation and leukorrhea, increase fertility, and ease pregnancy and childbirth problems are collectively termed *ching chan chi.*

Prophylaxis, diagnosis, and treatment of women's diseases are different from men's. Abnormal or irregular menstruation or amenorrhea yellow and red types. Problems associated with pregnancy include vomiting, fetal agitation, eclampsia, and edema. Labor may give rise to many kinds of medical problems, all of which are treated with these types of formulas.

Ching Chan Chi
Jing Chan Qi Gyneco-obstetric Formulas

* Dandelion Combination	*Pu-Kung-Ying-Tang* *Bu-Gung-Ying-Tang*
* Tang-kuei Formula	*Tang-kuei-San* *Dang-Gui-San*
* Tang-kuei & Evodia Combination	*Wen-Ching-Tang* *Wen-Jing-Tang*
* Tang-kuei & Gelatin Combination	*Chiung-Kuei-Chiao-Ai-Tang* *Qiong-Gu-E-Jiao-Tang*
* Tang-kuei & Ginger Combination	*Sheng-Hua-Tang* *Sheng-Hua-Tang*
* Tang-kuei & Peony Formula	*Tang-Kuei-Shao-Yao-San* *Dang-Gui-Shao-Yao-San*
* Tang-kuei & Parsley Combination	*An-Tai-Yin* *An-Tai-Yin*

Cinnamon & Persica Combination	*Che-Tsung-Yin* *Che-Zhong-Yin*
Chih-shih & Peony Combination	*Chih-Shih-Shao-Yao-San* *Zhi-Shi-Shao-Yao-San*
Cnidium & Rehmannia Combination	*Chiung-Kuei-Tiao-Hsieh-Yin* *Qiong-Gui-Tiao-Xie-Yin*
Persica & Eupolyphaga Combination	*Hsia-Yu-Hsieh-Tang* *Xia-Yu-Xue-Tang*
Biota & Achyranthes Formula	*Po-Tzu-Jen-Wan* *Bo-Zi-Ren-Wan*
Pteropus & Bulrush Formula	*Shih-Hsiao-San* *Shi-Xiao-San*

22
Tou Ma Chi
(痘麻劑 , Formulas for Childhood Diseases)

Formulas used for childhood diseases, especially measles, are termed *tou ma chi.*

Many sources have included this type of formula under the term *chieh piao chi.* With either measles or smallpox *Hsuan-tu-fa-piao-tang* (宣毒發表湯 , Cimicifuga and Peucedanum Combination) is often prescribed to encourage the toxin to come to the surface by means of acrid and cool herbs; *Sheng-ma-ko-ken-tang* (升麻葛根湯 , Cimicifuga and Pueraria Combination) is used to disperse the surface symptoms and speed maturation of the eruptions. In the event of pertussis (whooping cough), *San-ao-tang* (三拗湯 , Mahuang, Licorice, and Apricot Seed Combination) is used to clear the lungs and to ease muscle aching. *Ma-hsing-kan-shih-tang* (麻杏甘石湯 , Apricot Seed and Mahuang Combination) is used to cleanse the lungs by means of acrid and cool herbs. Some literature also includes acute and chronic infantile tetanus in this chapter.

Smallpox and measles are quarantined contagious diseases which must be reported to the authorities; these formulas must be used with care.

Tou Ma Chi
Tou Ma Qi Children's Formulas

Adenophora & Ophiopogon Combination	*Sha-Sheng-Mai-Tung-Tang* *Sha-Sheng-Mai-Tong-Tang*
Cimicifuga & Peucedanum Combination	*Hsuan-Tu-Fa-Piao-Tang* *Xuan-Tu-Fa-Biao-Tang*
Cimicifuga & Pueraria Combination	*Sheng-Ma-Ko-Ken-Tang* *Sheng-Ma-Ge-Gen-Tang*
Lepidium & Jujube Combination	*Ting-Li-Ta-Tsao-Hsieh-Fei-Tang* *Ting-Li-Da-Cao-Xie-Fei-Tang*
Mahuang, Licorice, & Apricot Seed Combination	*San-Ao-Tang* *San-Ao-Tang*

23
Ming Mu Chi
(明目劑, Eye Formulas)

Formulas that treat ocular diseases are called *ming mu chi.*

The development of ophthalmology as an independent branch of Chinese herbal medicine began during the Sung dynasty. Its therapeutics include internal, external, and surgical treatments. Internal treatment for eye ailments is based on the theoretical concept of there being a relationship between the eyes, the viscera, and the meridians. Localized pathological changes of the eyes are treated by external and surgical methods. The eye is divided into five regions, each called a *lun.* For example, the pupil is the water *lun* and the iris is the wind *lun.* Based on the diagnostic findings, an appropriate internal treatment is selected to adjust the visceral conditions or to attack injurious toxin. Then external treatment is coordinated to the internal treatment. Internal treatment is not only suitable for the eye diseases that arise from visceral or meridian disorders, but also is useful in treating eye diseases caused by epidemic infection or external injuries. Chinese herbal medicine often uses the wind-dispersing, fever-reducing, fire-purging, poison-detoxicating, or liver-supplementing, kidney-benefiting methods to effectively treat eye diseases.

Ming Mu Chi
Ming Mu Qi Eye Formulas

* Chrysanthemum Combination	*Tzu-Sheng-Ming-Mu-Tang* *Si-Sheng-Ming-Mu-Tang*
* Gardenia & Vitex Combination	*Hsi-Kan-Ming-Mu-Tang* *Xi-Gan-Ming-Mu-Tang*
Lycium, Chrysanthemum, & Rehmannia Formula	*Chi-Chu-Ti-Huang-Wan* *Ji-Zhu-Di-Huang-Wan*

24
Yung Yang Chi
(癰瘍劑 , Carbuncle-dermatosis Formulas)

Formulas that cleanse fever, detoxicate poisons, deflate swelling, soften hardening, and eliminate carbuncles are called *yung yang chi.*

Yung yang chi formulas treat internal and external carbuncles as well as various dermatoses. Internal factors include injuries caused by the seven emotions or by ingestion of acrid, hot, baked, or barbecued foods. External factors include the six excesses and all external wounds. Both internal and external factors can cause disharmony between the viscera and the skin, coagulation and stagnancy of *ch'i* and blood, and the occurrence of various carbuncular or dermatological changes. Treatment for these diseases includes internal and external methods. The internal method of treatment includes *tuo* (托 supporting), *pu* (補 supplementing), and *hsiao* (消 dissolving), depending on the stage of the disease. The external method acts directly on the lesion. Whatever method used, the formulas indicated are essentially antidotal, antiphlogistic, and fever-purging, and chiefly act to circulate and nourish the blood.

Descriptive terms are attached to the illustrative figure accompanying each formula. The terms are arranged clockwise beginning at the top of each figure.

Yung Yang Chi *Yung Yang Qi*	Formulas that 'cleanse' & detoxify fever poisons by nourishing and circulating blood

* Angelica & Mastic Combination	*Hsien-Fang-Huo-Ming-Yin* *Xian-Fang-Huo-Ming-Yin*
* Bupleurum & Schizonepeta Combination	*Shih-Wei-Pai-Tu-Tang* *Shi-Wei-Bai-Tu-Tang*
* Cimicifuga Combination	*I-Tzu-Tang* *I-Zi-Tang*
* Forsythia & Laminaria Combination	*San-Tsung-Kuei-Chien-Tang* *San-Zhong-Gui-Jian-Tang*

* Lithospermum & Oyster Shell Combination	*Tzu-Ken-Mu-Li-Tang* *Zi-Gen-Mu-Li-Tang*
* Lithospermum Ointment	*Tzu-Yun-Kao* *Zi-Yun-Gao*
* Ludwigia Formula	*Teng-Hua-Pai-Tu-San* *Teng-Hua-Pai-Tu-San*
* Rhubarb & Moutan Combination	*Ta-Huang-Mu-Tan-Pi-Tang* *Da-Huang-Mu-Tan-Pi-Tang*
* Schizonepeta & Forsythia Combination	*Ching-Chieh-Lien-Chiao-Tang* *Jing-Jie-Lian-Jiao-Tang*
* Schizonepeta & Siler Combination	*Ching-Fang-Pai-Tu-San* *Jing-Fang-Bai-Tu-San*
* Siler & Coix Combination	*Ching-Shang-Fang-Feng-Tang-Chia-I-Yi-Jen* *Jing-Shang-Fang-Feng-Tang-Jia-I-Yi-Ren*
* Tang-kuei & 8 Herb Formula	*Pa-Wei-Tai-Hsia-Fang* *Ba-Wei-Tai-Xia-Fang*
Platycodon Combination	*Chieh-Keng-Tang* *Jie-Geng-Tang*
Astragalus & Platycodon Formula	*Chien-Chin-Nei-Tuo-San* *Jian-Jin-Nei-Tuo-San*
Forsythia & Lonicera Formula	*Chih-Tou-Chung-I-Fang* *Zhi-Tou-Zhong-I-Fang*
Smilax & Akebia Combination	*Hsiang-Chun-Chieh-Tu-Chi* *Xiang-Zhun-Jie-Tu-Qi*
Coix, Aconite, & Thlaspi Formula	*I-Yi-Fu-Tzu-Pai-Chiang-San* *I-Yi-Fu-Zi-Bai-Xiang-San*
W.T.T.C.	*Lo-Shih-Shu* *Lo-Shi-Shu*
Platycodon & Chih-shih Formula	*Pai-Nung-San* *Bai-Nung-San*
Platycodon & Jujube Combination	*Pai-Nung-Tang* *Pai-Nung-Tang*
Eriocheir & Viper Formula	*Po-Chou-San* *Bo-Chou-San*
Moutan & Persica Combination	*Teng-Lung-Tang* *Teng-Long-Tang*

Dosage Forms and Uses of Chinese Herbal Formulas

After many generations, Chinese herbal physicians have developed many dosage forms, each of which has specific therapeutic characteristics. Here only the more commonly used forms are described.

Tang chi (湯劑 decoctions). Herbs are boiled with water and the liquid is called *tang chi,* for example *Ma-huang-tang* (麻黃湯 Mahuang Combination) and *Szu-ni-tang* (四逆湯 Aconite and G. L. Combination). Advantages of *tang chi* are easy absorption, fast action, and flexibility in adjusting the number or amount of the component herbs. Most acute conditions are treated with the *tang chi.*

San chi (散劑 powders). This dosage form is divided into internal and external powder. Internal powder is made by grinding all herbs into a powder that is taken with boiled water, rice gruel, or wine, as exemplified by *Wu-ling-san* (五苓散 Hoelen Five Herb Formula). External powder is likewise made by grinding all herbs into an extremely fine powder, but the powder is dusted on or applied to a wound, as exemplified by the surgical *Sheng-chi-san* (生肌散 Cuttlebone and Talc Formula).

Wan chi (丸劑 pill). This form is made by grinding all herbs into a very fine powder and then blending and kneading the powder with water, honey, flour paste, or rice paste, and forming pills. *Wan chi* is often used: (1) for debilitating diseases that require treatment over a long period of time, for example, *Liu-wei-ti-huang-wan* (六味地黃丸 Rehmannia Six Formula); (2) for blood extravasation or occlusion, and abdominal neoplasm or ascites that cannot be treated with a more powerful decoction, for example, *Ti-tang-wan* (抵當丸 Rhubarb and Leech Formula); (3) in combinations which require herbs with high toxicity that cannot be incorporated into a decoction, for example, *Pei-chi-wan* (備急丸 Rhubarb, Ginger, and Croton Formula); and (4) in combinations which require special herbs such as borneol and musk that are not suitable for a decoction preparation, for example, *Chih-pao-tan* (至寶丹 Rhinoceros and Succinum Formula).

Tiao chi (條劑 rods). A rod is made by gluing herb powder onto a thread or by rolling the herb powder into a rod which can then be inserted into a sore for the purpose of dissolving pus and removing fistulas.

Hsien chi (線劑 threads). A silk or cotton thread is immersed in a medicinal juice and boiled. Such a thread is used for tying up a fistula or polyp so that the latter withers and falls off.

Chin hsi chi (浸洗劑 washes). These are herbal decoctions used for soaking or washing either the whole or part of the body, for example, *Ku-sheng-tang* (苦參湯 Sophora Combination).

Hsun chi (薰劑 fumigants). The required herbs are burned and a lesion fumigated with the smoke, for example, realgar. In ancient times a boiling decoction of herbs was placed in a wooden keg. The patient sat on the keg above the decoction so that sweating could be induced by the fumes and heat.

Suan chi (栓劑 suppositories). A suppository is made the same way as a pill or tablet is made or by wrapping the herb powder in a silk or linen cloth. Suppositories are placed in the vagina for the treatment of abnormal leukorrhea or pudendal pruritus.

Tao fa (導法 guide-method or enema). Readily dissolvable or soluble herbs are formed into tablets and inserted in the anus. As the tablet dissolves, it lubricates the rectum and colon, making dry stool soft and easy to discharge. One such preparation is *Mi-chien-tao* (蜜煎導).

Kao chi (膏劑 unguents). This form is divided into internal and external types. Internal unguents are prepared by boiling sliced herbs repeatedly for a long time, then discarding the dregs. The solution is further condensed over a low fire and thickened into a salve by adding lumps of crystal sugar or honey. Such a dosage form can be taken over a long period of time and generally is the form in which most tonics are prepared. Hence tonics are also known as *kao tsu yao* (unguent tonics); an example is *Chuon-yu-kao* (瓊玉膏 Ginseng and Rehmannia Ointment). External unguents are ordinarily called plasters. They are made by boiling the herbs in oil, then discarding the dregs and adding cinnabar (red lead) and white vinegar. The ointment is finally heated and then spread over a piece of paper or cloth. The plaster so formed is placed on the surface of the body. They are often used for surgical carbunculosis or dermatosis, and for paralysis and aching due to winds and chills.

Tan chi (丹劑 pellets). *Tan chi* is also of two kinds, external and internal. *Tan chi*, a collective name, are mostly made of pure, refined, or very precious drugs. They are usually in fine powder form, sometimes bonded with glue or sticky herb juice. Examples are *Chih-pao-tan* (至寶丹 Rhinoceros and Succinum Formula), and internal, and *Hung-sheng-tan* (紅升丹 Cinnabar and Realgar Formula), an external.

Chiu chi (酒劑 elixirs). Also known as *yao chiu* (medicated liquor), elixirs are prepared by soaking the herbs in wine for a certain length of time or simmering them with wine in water, then removing the dregs. The remaining liquid is then drunk. One example of this form is *Hung-lan-hua-chiu* (紅藍花酒 Carthamus Wine), generally indicated for rheumatic paralysis and aching.

Yao lu (藥露 medicated essence). These essences are primarily distilled from fresh herbs. They have a light odor and bland taste and are commonly drunk for a summer medication; example: *Chin-yin-hua-lu* (金銀花露 Lonicera Essence).

Ting chi (錠劑), *ping chi* (餅劑 tablets, cakes). Herbs for tablets and cakes are pulverized into fine powders and admixed with some kind of mucilaginous juice. The mixture is kneaded and formed into tablets, *ting chi,* or small cakes, *ping chi.*

Of all these dosage forms, decoctions, pills, powders, unguents, and elixirs are the most frequently used. Based on the patient's condition, the length of use varies. Generally speaking though, if an herbal decoction is to be taken for an extended time in order to exert a healing action on the diseases in the upper warmer area, then the formula is taken after a meal. For diseases of the lower warmer, the medicine must be taken before meals to expedite the herbs in reaching the lower warmer. Tonics are taken on an empty stomach.

Appendix II

The List, Chinese Herbal Formulas of Sun Ten Products

Agent: Brion Corporation
12020 B, Centralia Road
Hawaiian Gardens, CA 90716
U. S. A.

PAGE	ITEM NO.	NAME
313	102	Aconite, Ginger, & Licorice Combination 四逆湯
100	106	Agastache Formula 藿香正氣散
511	108	Alisma Combination 澤瀉湯
535	110	Apricot & Linum Formula 麻子仁丸
46	112	Apricot & Perilla Formula 杏蘇散
230	116	Anemarrhena, Phellodendron, & Rehmannia Formula 知蘗八味丸
612	122	Angelica & Mastic Combination 仙方活命飲
169	128	Arctium Combination 清咽利膈湯
470	130	Areca Seed Combination 九檳吳茯湯
397	132	Areca & Evodia Combination 變製心氣飲
293	136	Astragalus Combination 黃耆建中湯
218	140	Astragalus & Atractylodes Combination 清暑益氣湯
523	144	Atractylodes Combination 越婢加朮湯
43	154	Minor Blue Dragon Combination 小青龍湯
343	158	Bupleurum Formula 抑肝散
112	160	Bupleurum & Chih-shih Formula 四逆散
117	162	Bupleurum and Cinnamon Combination 柴胡桂枝湯
85	164	Bupleurum, Cinnamon, and Ginger Combination 柴胡桂枝乾薑湯
340	166	Bupleurum and Dragon Bone Combination 柴胡加龍骨牡蠣湯
464	168	Bupleurum and Hoelen Combination 柴苓湯
87	170	Bupleurum and Peony Formula 加味逍遙散
35	172	Bupleurum and Pueraria Combination 柴葛解肌湯
160	174	Bupleurum & Rehmannia Combination 柴胡清肝湯
624	178	Bupleurum and Schizonepeta Combination 十味敗毒湯
543	180	Bupleurum and Scute Combination 柴陷湯
519	188	Capillaris Combination 茵陳蒿湯
521	190	Capillaris and Hoelen Formula 茵陳五苓散
104	192	Cardamon Combination 六和飲
366	196	Cardamon and Fennel Formula 安中散
600	202	Chrysanthemum Combination 滋腎明目湯
613	206	Cimicifuga Combination 乙字湯
63	212	Cinnamon Combination 桂枝湯
302	216	Cinnamon and Aconite Combination 桂枝加附子湯
305	218	Cinnamon, Aconite, & Ginger Combination 桂枝附子湯
450	220	Cinnamon and Anemarrhena Combination 桂枝芍藥知母湯
55	222	Cinnamon and Astragalus Combination 桂枝加黃耆湯
304	224	Cinnamon & Atractylodes Combination 桂枝加苓朮附湯
351	226	Cinnamon and Dragon Bone Combination 桂枝加龍骨牡蠣湯
179	228	Cinnamon Five Herb Combination 桂枝五物湯
306	230	Cinnamon & Ginseng Combination 桂枝人參湯
423	232	Cinnamon and Hoelen Formula 桂枝茯苓丸
60	234	Cinnamon and Peony Combination 桂枝加芍藥湯

* *Natural Healing with Chinese Herbs*

PAGE	ITEM NO.	NAME
561	636	Pinellia and Gastrodia Combination 半夏白朮天麻湯
110	640	Pinellia and Ginger Combination 生薑瀉心湯
254	642	Pinellia and Ginseng Six Combination 半瀉六君子湯
487	646	Minor Pinellia and Hoelen Combination 小半夏加茯苓湯
103	650	Pinellia and Licorice Combination 甘草瀉心湯
395	656	Pinellia and Magnolia Combination 半夏厚朴湯
548	670	Platycodon and Fritillary Combination 清肺湯
	674	Platycodon and Gypsum Combination 桔梗石膏湯
472	684	Polyporus Combination 豬苓湯
51	690	Pueraria Combination 葛根湯
122	694	Pueraria, Coptis, and Scute Combination 葛根黃連黃芩湯
50	700	Pueraria and Magnolia Combination 葛根湯加川芎辛夷
37	706	Pueraria Nasal Combination 清鼻湯
245	720	Rehmannia Six Formula 六味地黃
250	722	Rehmannia Eight Formula 八味地黃
626	734	Rhubarb and Moutan Combination 大黃牡丹皮湯
607	744	Schizonepeta and Forsythia Combination 荆芥連翹湯
609	748	Schizonepeta and Siler Formula 荆防敗毒散
271	754	Scute Combination 滋腎通耳湯
(565)*	764	Siler Combination 清上防風湯
610	768	Siler & Coix Combination 清上防風湯加薏苡仁
119	778	Siler and Platycodon Formula 防風通聖散
477	788	Stephania and Astragalus Combination 防己黃耆湯
500	790	Stephania and Ginseng Combination 木防己湯
177	794	Sweet Combination 甘露飲
432	808	Tang-kuei Four Combination 四物湯
618	810	Tang-kuei and Eight Herb Formula 八味帶下方散
402	814	Tang-kuei Sixteen Herb Combination 十六味流氣飲
506	818	Tang-kuei & Anemarrhena Combination 當歸拈痛湯
572	820	Tang-kuei & Parsley Combination 安胎飲
445	822	Tang-kuei and Arctium Formula 消風散
94	826	Tang-kuei & Bupleurum Formula 逍遙散
588	830	Tang-kuei and Evodia Combination 溫經湯
319	834	Tang-kuei, Evodia, and Ginger Combination 當歸四逆加吳茱萸生薑湯
415	838	Tang-kuei and Gambir Combination 七物降下湯
439	842	Tang-kuei and Gardenia Combination 溫清飲
576	844	Tang-kuei and Gelatin Combination 芎歸膠艾湯
583	846	Tang-kuei and Ginger Combination 生化湯
248	848	Tang-kuei & Ginseng 8 Combination 八珍湯
130	854	Tang-kuei & Magnolia Formula 五積散

* *Natural Healing with Chinese Herbs*

PAGE	ITEM NO.	NAME
585	860	Tang kuei and Peony Formula 當歸芍藥散
459	874	Tuhuo and Vaeicum Combination 獨活寄生湯
278	930	Vitality Combination 眞武湯
617	960	W.T.T.C. 樂適舒
196	970	Xanthium Formula 蒼耳散
355	980	Zizyphus Combination 酸棗仁湯
634	999	Lithospermum Ointment 紫雲膏
	1001	American Ginseng Powder (100% pure)

Formula Index

(C) = Commonly Used Chinese Herb Formulas with Illustrations
(N) = Natural Healing with Chinese Herbs

A

B

D

H

I

N

O

P

R

S

T

Abbreviations

abd., abdom.	:	abdominal	P	:	Pulse
Comb.	:	Combination	pt	:	patient
esp.	:	especially	S. I.	:	small intestine
freq.	:	frequent	sp	:	spleen
he	:	heart	spont.	:	spontaneous
ki	:	kidney	st	:	stomach
L. I.	:	large intestine	T	:	Tongue
lu	:	lung	Tx	:	treatment
lv	:	liver	$\bar{\bar{w}}$	:	with

Other Publications of the Oriental Healing Arts Institute

CHIN KUEI YAO LUEH

The first English translation of the Chinese medical classic **Chin Kuei Yao lueh** (Prescriptions from the Golden Chamber) provides a wealth of information on the etiology and treatment of internal disease. As a primary source, the book also covers surgery, pregnancy, and dietary rules of the ancient Chinese and gives step-by-step instructions for the preparation of 205 herbal formulas still used today by traditional Chinese physicians, "barefoot doctors" in China, and **Kanpō** practitioners in Japan. Anyone interested in medical history, folk medicine, or sinology will find the material fascinating and thought provoking. Scholars of Chinese culture will especially appreciate the perspective that unfolds in the historical commentaries found in the Foreward, Introduction, and Preface. *Hsu, Hong-yen, Ph.D. 1983. 240 pages. Paper $12.00. Hardback $15.00*

CHINESE HERB MEDICINE AND THERAPY REVISED EDITION

The popularity of the first edition of **Chinese Herb Medicine and Therapy**, in spite of its rough English, inspired the staff of the Oriental Healing Arts Institute to revise the much-needed material and smooth out its grammar. The revised text, a major departure from the original, is broad in scope and incorporates all the major principles and theory underlying Chinese medicine: methods of diagnosis, principles of treatment, medical theory on selected problems, properties of herbs, categorized prescriptions, in-depth analyses of 68 formulas, descriptions of over 100 commonly used herbs, and extensive indexes for easy reference. A comprehensive introduction to Chinese herbal medicine, this book will serve as a substantive source for anyone interested in alternative therapies. *Hsu, Hong-yen, Ph.D., and Peacher, William G., M.D., 1983. Oversize. 317 pages. Illustrated. Paper $12.00. Hardback $15.00*

HOW TO TREAT YOURSELF WITH CHINESE HERBS

This handbook explains in clear and concise language how the Chinese use herbs to achieve good health. The first section reviews 14 categories of chronic and acute illnesses and their therapies. The following sections include a discussion of 95 herbs and 128 formulas, their uses and healing properties. *Hsu, Hong-yen, Ph.D., 1980. Paper. 296 pages. Illustrated $5.95*

COMMONLY USED CHINESE HERB FORMULAS WITH ILLUSTRATIONS

An extensive compilation of the herbal formulas commonly prescribed by physicians who follow the Chinese herbal tradition. Twenty-four categories of formulas are presented according to their pharmaceutical action: emetics, purgatives, anthelmintics, *ch'i* formulas, sedatives, etc. Included in each formula's entry are its ingredients, indications, and discriminatory symptoms, plus an anatomical diagram showing the targets of treatment. *Hsu, Hong-yen, Ph.D., & Hsu, Chau-shin, Ph.D., 1982. 671 pages. Illustrated. Paper $19.95. Hardback $25.00*

THE WAY TO GOOD HEALTH WITH CHINESE HERBS

A concise and easily understood guidebook to Chinese herbal medicine. **The Way to Good Health with Chinese Herbs** covers diet therapy for various problems and outlines herbal formulas for specific diseases. Symptoms are clearly described for each formula and the herbs making up the formulas are listed. For easy reference, the contents are arranged in alphabetical order. Once again, Dr. Hsu brings us another valuable reference work. For the first time, some of the information known and used by the Chinese for centuries is available to the English reader. In particular, Dr. Hsu introduces diet therapy, an integral part of Chinese medicine and culture. **The Way to Good Health with Chinese Herbs** definitely expands our knowledge in the field of alternative therapy. *Hsu, Hong-yen, Ph.D. 1983. Paper. 230 pages. $7.00*

Available by mail from. . . . .

ORIENTAL HEALING ARTS INSTITUTE
1945 PALO VERDE AVE. SUITE 208
LONG BEACH, CALIFORNIA 90815

(Price includes postage and handling. California residents please add 6.5% sales tax.)